SACRED
RELATIONSHIPS

"This latest work is a true guidebook for those on the mystical and conscious path of divine loving. The authors seamlessly bring together deep esoteric wisdom with practical application for those on the path—whether single or coupled. The practices, with expanded wisdom and spiritual meaning, allow those called to go deeper into heart and soul-centered loving. A must-read for divine lovers everywhere!"

HEATHER STRANG, SPIRITUAL TEACHER AND
AUTHOR OF *THE QUEST: A TALE OF DESIRE & MAGIC*

"This amazing book provides profound insight into the new paradigm of relationships in a way I've never seen before. The authors expertly navigate through the often confounding subject to reach the core of the Divine Human experience. Through these 72 pearls of wisdom you'll discover your own relationship with divinity and your perfect partner."

JAMES F. TWYMAN, PEACE TROUBADOUR
AND AUTHOR OF *THE MOSES CODE*

SACRED
RELATIONSHIPS

"This latest work is a true guidebook for those on the mystical and conscious path of divine loving. The authors seamlessly bring together deep esoteric wisdom with practical application for those on the path—whether single or coupled. The practices, with expanded wisdom and spiritual meaning, allow those called to go deeper into the art and soul-centered loving. A must-read for divine lovers everywhere!"

—HEATHER STRANG, SPIRITUAL TEACHER AND
AUTHOR OF THE QUEST: TANTRA OF DANCE & ALICE

"This amazing book provides profound insight into the new paradigm of relationships in a way I've never seen before. The authors expertly navigate through the often confounding subject to reach the core of the Divine Human experience. Through these 72 pearls of wisdom you'll discover your own relationship with divinity and your perfect partner."

—JAMES F. TWYMAN, PEACE TROUBADOUR
AND AUTHOR OF THE MOSES CODE

SACRED
RELATIONSHIPS

The Practice of
Intimate Erotic Love

ANAIYA SOPHIA
and
PADMA AON PRAKASHA

Destiny Books
Rochester, Vermont • Toronto, Canada

Destiny Books
One Park Street
Rochester, Vermont 05767
www.DestinyBooks.com

Destiny Books is a division of Inner Traditions International

Library of Congress Cataloging-in-Publication Data
Names: Sophia, Anaiya, 1969– author. | Prakasha, Padma Aon, author.
    Title: Sacred relationships : the practice of intimate erotic love / Anaiya Sophia,
Padma Aon Prakasha.
Description: Rochester, Vermont : Destiny Books, 2017. | Includes index.
    Identifiers: LCCN 2016021137 (print) | LCCN 2016053312 (e-book) |
    ISBN 9781620555491 (paperback) | ISBN 9781620555507 (e-book)
Subjects: LCSH: Sex instruction. | Sex—Religious aspects. | Love—Religious
    aspects. | BISAC: SELF-HELP / Sexual Instruction. | HEALTH & FITNESS
    / Sexuality.
Classification: LCC HQ56 .S667 2017 (print) | LCC HQ56 (e-book) |
    DDC 613.9071—dc23
LC record available at https://lccn.loc.gov/2016021137

Printed and bound in the United States

10 9 8 7 6 5 4 3

Text design and layout by Virginia Scott Bowman
This book was typeset in Garamond Premier Pro with Hypatia Sans used as the
    display typeface
Artwork by Cathy Hilton, www.cathyhiltonartisan.co.uk

To send correspondence to the authors of this book, mail a first-class letter to the
authors c/o Inner Traditions • Bear & Company, One Park Street, Rochester, VT
05767, and we will forward the communication, or contact the authors directly at
www.anaiyasophia.com or **www.padmaaon.com**.

Dedicated to Our Beloved

CONTENTS

BOOK OF WISDOM
✦
ATTRIBUTES OF THE DIVINE FEMININE

BOOK OF TRUTH
✦
ATTRIBUTES OF THE DIVINE MASCULINE

BOOK OF ALCHEMY
✦
ATTRIBUTES OF DIVINE MARRIAGE

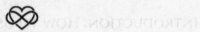

ALCHEMICAL BODY PRACTICES

ACKNOWLEDGMENTS

From Anaiya: To my parents, Dinah and Patrick Cuddihy, thank you for taking me to Sacré-Coeur in Paris—upon whose steps I saw the face of love—when I was seven years old. Thank you both so deeply for birthing within me this inextinguishable fire of love and for bringing me into this world in the first place.

To my passionate contributor and editor, Jenna Paulden, who always shows up, more and deeper, utterly committed to the path and to our journey as Sisters within the Feminine Christ, thank you for contributing your own Pearls of Wisdom to this book—Communication, Gratitude, Listening, and Sovereignty.

To my dear friend and fellow pilgrim Cathy Hilton, who almost overnight miraculously produced all the illustrations for this book, thank you.

Thank you to Padma, for stepping in and birthing the Divine Masculine voice for this book. Without you, the book could not have been completed.

To my mentor Andrew Harvey, for being the compelling force that takes me beyond myself.

To Jon Graham, Meghan MacLean, Manzanita Carpenter, and the team at Inner Traditions, who supported the birth of this book during a time of tremendous personal growth and expansion, thank you for making this process so graceful. It is always a delight to work with you all. Thank you for being our publishers and for continuing to support the birth of our message into the world and into the hearts of many.

From Padma: Shekinah Zorensky—thank you, dear sister and friend of my heart, for your support and for your help with writing about the Mother.

Aina Greta—thank you for all you do and for your willingness, love, and care.

I thank Anaiya Sophia for her trust, desire, and openness in inviting me to write this book with her.

May you all know how deeply you have touched us and how this touch reverberates throughout the entire Cosmos.

PREFACE

By Anaiya Sophia

The core mystery of this era is the birth of the Divine Human. A being that has fused together within himself or herself all the opposites: light and dark, body and soul, transcendent and immanent, masculine and feminine.

The wisdom gathered in this book has been drawn together in a myriad of ways, ranging from deep mystical insights, initiations, and relationships to the experience of streetwise common sense. These Pearls of Wisdom are the fruits of our personal experiences journeying into Sacred Relationship and the divinization process that the new paradigm brings.

Sacred Relationships illuminates many of the obstacles and grace-filled ecstasies that came as one important relationship in our lives ended and the seeds of other ones were sown. This book also includes contributions and quotes from other midwives and sacred warriors on the path of Sacred Relationship.

Trust, holy desire, and humility allow one to step off the cliff and risk all. Inevitably this book shall speak the loudest to those who have these essential qualities or want to develop them. For us, Sacred Relationship is the place where we have grown more radically than in any other area of life. We have experienced the beloved relationship, the parent-child relationship, the mentor-apprentice model, and even the new paradigm community collective relationship! However, it is always in Sacred Relationship where the rubber hits the road and our edges are softened. Some of this softening and resultant growth has been difficult and painful, but in the end it has always served to open our hearts.

Sacred Relationships is a road map and oracular prayer. It brings forth mystical teachings that can reactivate our primordial, often forgotten voice, our pure sexual expression in harmony with the Divine, and the presence of deep-rooted wisdom within us. By reintegrating wisdom into relationship, a fully awakened couple is born. This divine pair has the power to dissolve the patterns, beliefs, and behaviors that remain entrenched within the old paradigm. Furthermore, they create a template of the new paradigm with their clear-feeling vision. These beings have reclaimed their power and are not afraid to use it to let go and create anew. With their throne of sovereignty reinstated, all psychic entrapments and emotional obstacles simply fall away, making space for creation to enter.

This book is a rich resource of mystical feminine wisdom and transcendent masculine consciousness, and it births a practical, realistic path to bring women and men together as one. Within the core of all divine unions, we discover the true kernel of lasting transformation. Within the womb of woman and the *hara,* an energetic region in the lower torso, of man lives a resource that can activate the forces designed for the complete transfiguration from human to divine. This force is known as Shakti, a brimming, teeming life force that helplessly flows toward deeper consciousness (Shiva). We cannot prevent Shakti from merging with Shiva; this is the Divine Marriage in action.

To facilitate the return to our original wholeness, we must take some essential healing steps. Before we can open to the full sacredness of divine union, we must melt all shadowy forms of body hatred, sexual shame, emotional wounding, and gender animosity. The teachings within this book are devoted to such a process. Lovingly imbued with the tenderness of the feminine and precisely instructed by the awareness of the masculine, these words, transmissions, and practices are designed to penetrate at the deepest level and guide you toward the gnosis, or direct knowing, within your own soul.

Not only does sexuality require a completely conscious transfiguration, it also calls for a transformation of what is held within one's heart and psychology. Our ability to love at the level of holiness has become enshrouded by layers of fortified protection. Hidden in the intricate catacombs of the mind, our personality continues to harbor thoughts of fear, separation, and isolation.

All of this has to be offered up to the high altar of love. God's love. And one of the most important things that we have learned about this love is that it requires our trust. The two go hand in hand. We need to trust ourselves. We need to trust our partners. And we need to trust God. We need to trust in love and the process—completely—all the way to the end of the road. This may lead to God knows where, but our faith in the journey will bring about its conscious completion. Lack of trust in any of these areas undermines our relationships and makes it impossible for us to penetrate and heal the veil of fear that separates us from one another.

Trust is based on a willingness to explore and an ability to evolve. We simply cannot trust a person we don't respect, don't accept, and don't desire to be vulnerable with. The attempt to do so is one of the most frustrating aspects of relationship. Without trust, love is infantile and selfish. Indeed, to call it love is to misname it and trivialize it. At the beginning stages of relationship, we must ask ourselves these questions in the cool, still center of our being. *Do I respect this person? Do I accept this person? Do I want to be vulnerable with this person? Does this person have a true and real center? Does this person have what it takes to hold me and all that I am as well as the mystery of all that I shall become?*

If we really choose the path of Sacred Relationship and desire deeply to be transformed, then we have to embrace our partners fully. We must be willing to let our partners be just as they are. That means no fixing, no saving, no remaking of our partners to fit our idealized vision or anyone else's—including those of our parents or our friends. This doesn't mean that we think our partners are perfect. We simply see them as they are, with all imperfections, and we accept those as part of the total picture.

The inability to see and hold our partners' wholeness is symptomatic of our inability to see and hold our own. Most of us have deeply divided relationships with ourselves—and these divisions arise in double time once we have committed to Sacred Relationship. This internal fragmentation plays out as neurotic thoughts and emotions and ambivalent behavior toward our partners. Yet, at the molten core of divine union is wholeness. Wholeness within oneself extends to wholeness with the other.

This doesn't mean that we *think* we are whole, because there are certainly times when it *feels* that we are not. Wholeness comes when a being has a palpable connection to God. In any challenge this being does not fall apart or get hysterical, but instead turns inward and calmly moves in the direction of the One who bestows that wholeness. In that peaceful and benevolent state, grace enters.

This internal process has to be the backbone of your spiritual practice. It connects you with your essence, giving you the ability to endure this transformational process. When couples lack inner confidence, have no real faith in a greater source of wisdom than their human minds, and are ambivalent toward one another, how on Earth can this internal shift ever take place? Without a palpable connection to the Divine and each one's inner wholeness, this great journey together will not come to fruition. It takes not only intention and desire but also practice.

We are living in a time on our planet when we are being called to reach deep inside to find the courage for undertaking an incredibly challenging and amazing act of creation—the birth of the Divine Human. This genesis is happening right now, all over the world, not just in humankind, but within all of life and Earth herself. We believe this shift is the answer to our existential crisis as well as the deepest meaning of it. The birth of the Divine Human is, in fact, the key to our evolutionary destiny.

Unless we call forth and embody the commitment to stay as humble as possible, none of us will successfully enter the firestorm of this great evolutionary movement that is being directed straight toward humanity from the heart of Godhead. We have to commit to a daily infusion of prayer, love, humility, openness, and truth on every level of our being. Without daily and consistent replenishment, our spiritual backbone may break. Let us not underestimate the gravity of what we are embarking upon.

We are asking to be made divine, to be restored to our original wholeness. We are asking to fuse the inherent holiness of our soul with our human self, thus creating a divinized human—an archetype for the awakened, co-creative beings of the new Earth. God's eyes have *always* seen us as holy and whole. Yet for millennia the fragmented human emotional state and ego have trained us to believe in the illusion of separation. Now is the time for us to humbly, yet powerfully, step into our sovereignty and see ourselves truly as we are—divine reflections of God. In fact, we are asking to see the world *with* the eyes of God and bless all we see.

Humility is the only virtue that will allow us to stay empty. No matter what we seem to achieve along the way, unless we continually empty ourselves, we cannot be filled with divine love. Unless we stay empty, we cannot be continually taken forward. Only when we bend our knees in adoration, gratitude, and surrender will this fundamental yet immense transfiguration be integrated. Only in humility and openness will it become real.

Dearest Readers, may the seeds of this wisdom be planted in your heart and blossom into your life. May you drink deeply from this well and quench your thirst for love and truth. May you forgive and heal. May you come into the fullness of your union. May you experience your divinity through the grace of Sacred Relationship. And may we all support, love, and take care of one another along the way. And so, on that exquisite note, I wish to give thanks to all the lovers and friends who have helped me to grow, to love, and to trust the truth.

IN LOVE,
ANAIYA SOPHIA

The highest form of spiritual practice, for those of us who aspire to create Heaven on Earth, is our relationships with one another.

ANDREW COHEN,
"SPIRITUAL PRACTICE IS SPIRIT LIVED"

PREFACE

By Padma Aon Prakasha

Sacred Relationship involves two individual souls and God. The first step is that each individual has a direct, soul-felt, feeling relationship to Mother-Father God. In this sacred trinity of self, the beloved, and Mother-Father God, the relationship becomes an alchemical container of transformation. Sacred Relationships are partnerships overlighted by God, fueled by each soul's deep longing and knowing that the soul is here on Earth to experience this as part of its divine design.

Our feelings make us who we are and define our soul. They are our vital, living connection to the Divine—how we communicate with God and directly to another soul. Experiencing all our feelings by moving through them and releasing them allows us to become truly alive in a state of loving peace, care, joy, and contentment.

Sacred Relationships are the initiatory temples of today. They are where we learn to truly feel, give, and receive. They bring us to the heights of bliss and plummet us into the depths of our pain. They are our boon and bane.

Sacred Relationship entails the unifying of sexual energy and your emotions with God. These are two of the most challenging areas for modern-day humanity. God has been relegated to an anachronism and tool of fear-inducing religious beliefs; God as an entity has been reduced to a field, rather than a personal, living soul whom we all have access to directly through our hearts and who responds to us and loves us perfectly.

Our emotions are misunderstood, judged, denied, and prematurely transcended in favor of a "higher" spirituality that sees emotions as something to be witnessed and avoided, rather than something to embrace and develop into fullness through humility and vulnerability. Both are included on the beloved path, for it is only through embracing our emotions that we realize union.

Sexuality is still largely repressed, bought and sold as a commodity, and feared because of its awesome power to take us out of the mundane and into the extraordinary. Indeed, as American spiritual teacher Andrew Cohen shares, "Many people feel so overwhelmed by the power of the sexual impulse that instead of it really being empowering, they often feel victimized by it, feeling that *the power of this force is stronger than me.* Unless we get to a point where we know that who we are is stronger than that primal impulse, we are never going to be able to embrace and express it in any kind of spiritual manner."*

All these enormous powers unify in Sacred Union. It is the greatest challenge and most enormous fulfillment a human being can undertake, as nothing is left out, all is included, and everything within one's self has to be explored. This is why few people, until now, truly could set out on this journey.

In divine relating a man becomes a King and a woman becomes a Queen. Through the container and furnace of this relationship, divine men and divine women are forged. The Divine Masculine and Divine Feminine are not created in isolation. Kings and Queens create each other; they are not born like that. For a man to become a King, he needs to be one with his inner feminine. For a woman to become a Queen, she needs to be one with her inner masculine. When this inner state is reflected in outer relationships, then the Queendom of Heaven is here on Earth.

Sexuality that includes loving feeling forms a deep part of our most

---

*This is an excerpt from Andrew Cohen's magazine *What Is Enlightenment?* (later titled *EnlightenNext*).

blissful, ecstatic states. God loves sex and sexual expression, and the creation of our own soul is the result of God's sexual expression. One of the primary purposes of our physical and spiritual bodies' designs is sexual expression. Without it we are incomplete, for avoidance of sexual power causes denials and pain within the soul, preventing spiritual development.

Sexuality is a core soul quality that when developed in union with love, enables you to have a loving connection with yourself and with your partner and to deepen a pure connection with God.

Sexuality begins with a presumption of opposites. Opposites have to unite to experience union. If you take two unenlightened people and put them together with the idea that they need each other to experience spiritual union or fulfillment, problems arise. They will think this relationship is going to give them an experience of intimacy with life, with self, with other, and with Spirit or God. And maybe it will. But because God or Spirit has not been found within, we can tend to project our craving for spiritual union onto our romantic relationships, and make them the cause for our own suffering.

A particular illusion suffered by many on the Spiritual Path today is the projection of their idealized partner or soul mate onto someone who is not that. You project your unresolved needs, wounds, and Hollywood expectations onto another, hoping he or she will make it all better for you. The concept of soul mates is manna from heaven for those who are emotionally wounded and seek wholeness outside of themselves.

Honesty and humility are the only ways out of this illusion, freeing both of you from the inevitable chain of unmet expectations, demands, and resentments that will arise from this. Projecting your soul-mate feelings toward other people will never work and will inevitably end badly.

Most relationships at this time on Earth are wounded attractions: one wound in one person resonates to the other. The hole in one person attracts a hook in another and vice versa. The hole is a wound, an opening in one partner; the hook in the other, like a tentacle, grasps instantly at this hole. They meet, and a potent charge is felt, which many misinterpret as love.

While this attraction feels powerful, it is based on compatible emotional injuries and is karmic in nature. It is there for both people to identify and heal from. If seen and dealt with consciously, this type of relationship can lead to healing, and once the healing is complete, the stage is set for you to meet your true soul mate.

Essentially, what you want from the other person is what you are unwilling to feel within yourself. No one can heal you, only your desire, humility, and awareness can—with the help of God. Others can support you, but not do it for you. Once you feel and accept the truth of yourself, only then can truth and love bloom, free from belief, projection, and need.

> *If you continue to pursue the goal of salvation through a relationship, you will be disillusioned again and again. But if you accept that the relationship is here to make you conscious instead of happy, then the relationship will offer you salvation, and you will be aligning yourself with the higher consciousness that wants to be born into this world. For those who hold to the old patterns, there will be increasing pain, violence, confusion, and madness.*
>
> ECKHART TOLLE,
> *PRACTICING THE POWER OF NOW*

Pursuing salvation through another, in any way, will lead to experiences where you are drawn into your worst fears. To know yourself in this darkness is an opportunity to heal those parts of yourself that you are unwilling to experience. In the other extreme, those who live lives of cool emotional detachment often do so when they are unable or unwilling to face their fears.

The biggest problem in relationships is what we neglect to include. What we all yearn for, what we all miss and secretly desire, and what we mistakenly try to get from one another is divine love and God. We look for this form of love from another person, but we will never, ever, get it. It is our human needs and wounds that make us feel that human love alone is our salvation. We think that human love will make everything right in our lives, that it will make everything better. Human love and sex will never satisfy us, because what we are really searching for is divine love directly from God. Instead, we place another person before God as our holy grail, and he or she becomes a substitute that will never fulfill our deepest desires or heal our wounds.

The paradox is that when both partners place God first, in feeling and desire, the love *within* each partner and the love *between* them magnifies tremendously, as there is no longer any need to get this love from the other person. There are no more substitutes; there is just a desire to give and share more truth in love.

In a human sexual relationship with God installed as the center and unmoving fulcrum, God helps to guide the relationship. With God installed as the primary force, human relationships and sexuality bloom to their full potential of human love and divine love merging in bliss, pleasure, play, trust, gratitude, and honest, humble interactions.

In this divine relating sexuality, a burning yearning for God, and the feeling depths of the human soul are brought together. This is not about two souls merging together. In Sacred Relationship the purpose is for each soul to merge with God, first and foremost.

The soul close to God has no desperate needs from his or her partner because God fulfills him or her. If you are deeply committed to the Divine, this is reflected in every aspect of your life. Union with God is not something done alone in your prayer room; it is a way of life. God lives in the bedroom too. Everything has to reflect this union, including your sexuality and the one you share your life and bed with.

Dearest Readers, may these Pearls of Wisdom be seeded in your heart and blossom in your life. May you dive deeply into the truth of love, human and Divine, and emerge humbled, powerful, loving, and wise. May we all enjoy the ecstasy and freedom that holy desire brings to us as we emerge into the Divine Child of God that we are destined to be.

PADMA AON PRAKASHA

INTRODUCTION

HOW TO USE THIS BOOK

The wisdom teachings found within this book can be explored in a variety of ways. You may open the book, start at the beginning, and read it in a linear way. Or you might like to use the book as an oracle, randomly opening a page in response to a question. Of course, you are always invited to invent new ways of using this book. Just remember, the most important thing is to approach *Sacred Relationships* with an open heart, see where it resonates with your soul's wisdom—and enjoy the journey!

Sacred Relationships contains sixty-six Pearls of Wisdom and six alchemical body practices for a total of seventy-two keys to help you birth divinity into your own human form. They are transmissions designed to awaken within you ways to explore and feel into your true self. As you read and absorb the teachings in this book, an inner adventure will unfold, and it will reveal the path at your own pace, cultivating the expansion of trust and consciousness along the way. This book was created in the spirit of mystical revelation; its intent is to initiate in the reader experiences of gnosis, or direct knowing.

Before we begin we must first understand that the terms *masculine* and *feminine* do not refer to just the male and female forms. Sacred Marriage is the union of these two forces in our own psyche and human identity. Each and every single one of us has an inner masculine and feminine expression and perception that we have to learn from and

1

unite within us. Men have to experience, live, and integrate both the feminine and masculine qualities to become a King, and women have to experience, live, and integrate both the masculine and feminine qualities to become a Queen. We are both masculine and feminine and neither at different times, for this union creates something new. The masculine within us is the clear voice of order, the courage to stand up and speak out, the ability to focus, and the protector of innocence and freedom. The feminine within us is the profound desire to love, the celebration of the deep and sacred, the ability to feel and intimately connect, and the nurturer of community, friendship, and Nature.

Unified they create the Divine Human.

Please also note that the Divine, or God, is also composed of both masculine and feminine and is referred to throughout this book as both. Sometimes we use God/Father/him, sometimes Goddess/Mother/her, and other times we use Mother-Father/God-Goddess/him-her (among other names). Know that they are all one, the One, the Divine.

Sacred Relationships is a codebook containing consciousness keys to seed the new paradigm in a way that can be received, integrated, and acted upon. To apply these keys directly to your life, you need to know which ones apply specifically to you at any given time. If you use the book as an oracle, the moment you open to a particular page with prayerful intent and a clear question you will receive correct guidance. You are then invited to contemplate the wisdom therein, and act upon it using the prayers and practices for that particular Pearl of Wisdom. If you are reading the book from cover to cover, you may slowly digest each key, one at a time. Read with awareness, and allow the deeper meanings between the lines to come to you in dream, vision, self-inquiry, meditation, and prayer. You may also simply go about your day, holding the intention to receive the significance of any particular Pearl of Wisdom that you are working on. Take your time and stay present.

No matter how you choose to go about it, ensure that you eventually contemplate each of the seventy-two pearls and alchemical practices. Every pearl and practice is part of the entire transmission. Each one contains a unique message with a layered meaning, and each message takes time to absorb. Bear in mind that contemplating is far more than simply thinking about something. It is the direct absorption of wisdom at a physical, emotional, psychological, and spiritual level—and it leads to action.

One of the ways to open to the hidden aspects of this wisdom is to simply ask for the deeper meaning to arise in your consciousness. By pondering, wondering, and gently allowing, you will be able to see beyond the habitual patterns of the old paradigm and begin to grow toward something new. At such times the pearl you find yourself reading—whether randomly revealed or linearly followed—will highlight the hidden essence of a current issue. It may seem uncanny to the old paradigm mind, but the Universe acts with exactly this kind of synchronicity as you align with the new paradigm. *Ask and it shall be given!*

If you are experiencing a shadow state or working through difficult and painful emotions, or if you find yourself on the receiving end of negative behavior, close your eyes and hold the book to your heart. Take the time to pray for a deeper, more compassionate understanding of what is needed within yourself and your relationship. Affirm that whatever it is, it will allow you to grow to the next level. Keeping your eyes closed, intuitively feel a certain page. There you will have it—the wisdom needed at that very moment in order to grow in love. Trust it.

However you choose to read the book, our intention is that it may be a companion for you—one that offers support, deep insight, and a steady, loving handrail during those inevitable moments of doubt, despair, and confusion. We offer a deep prayer that *Sacred Relationships* becomes your roadmap out of the old paradigm and into the new.

And so it is!

BOOK OF WISDOM
Attributes of the Divine Feminine

I Am: Pure Love.

I Am Wisdom, benevolently flowing in Divine Elegance, Source of Comfort, Full of Compassion and Passion. I Am Breath.

I Am Sovereign, Queen who serves all, Mother, Lover, Divine Woman.

I Am a Yoni of Love.

I Am Benevolent and Virginal, a Rhythmic, Primordial Power of Joy.

I Am the Compassion of Woman as the Daughter of My Mother, Tantric Muse of Embodied Love and Transmuting Elegance: I Am Embodiment.

The wisdom of the Divine Feminine, together with the mythological and mystical tradition that attends it, is returning to consciousness. This wisdom reconnects us to a dimension of the instinctual soul that has been shut away, like Sleeping Beauty, behind a hedge of thorns. The power and luminosity of the Divine Feminine are needed now—to arouse the will, inhabit the body, and imbue our existence with an abundance of energy that inspires us to act on behalf of life. She calls for us to restore wholeness and co-creative awareness to our image of God, our image of relationship, and our image of ourselves. The return of the Divine Feminine is awakening humanity to a new ethic of responsibility, focused beyond our individual concerns toward the needs of the planet and the birth of the new paradigm.

BENEVOLENCE

Benevolence—well-meaning kindness, decency, and kind-heartedness

Benevolence is silent goodwill. It is like the sun shining on hard ground, softening the earth, melting the ice, but with no design or intention to affect things. It is the state of uninterrupted naturalness, which is why it works, because the ground feels no debt to the sun. In the same way, to be on the receiving end of benevolence is to receive something for which there is no return. No pressure to respond creates a natural, easy response.

Benevolence is a state of being, reliant on itself alone. It has nothing to do with feelings of mercy or preference. It offers nothing specific, but everyone is drawn to it. It answers no questions, but it enables you to think. It teaches nothing, but because of it you can learn.

To be benevolent is to have forged a link with an unbroken source of kindness so strong that even the interruptions of life cannot block that constant refueling. However dry life is, the tide keeps turning again and again, always. And in the moments just before turning, when life has taken you to the limits, you just know that you're on the brink of a great inflow, and so you stay quiet, acknowledging temporary emptiness—yet only as a prelude.

The word *benevolence* comes from the Latin roots *bene*, "well," and *velle*, "to wish"—"to wish well." Benevolence is not only the desire to bring kindness to another, it is also the *ability* to do so. Benevolence is kindness in action—extending goodness to one's self, to others, and to life. Benevolence springs from a deep place of gentleness and compassion within.

Holy Prayer

✦

Beloved Mother Father God, help me to see where I am being harmful despite my best intentions, and allow me to soften. Help me to see where I am being unkind, and allow me to become compassionate. Grant me the humility to be able to see the true nature of my thoughts, words, and actions, and grace me the purity to be able to uplift them. On this day, beloved Benevolent One, encourage me to extend well-meaning kindness to all. Amen.

⑤ Sacred Action

Take some deep breaths and then ask yourself these sacred questions while looking in a mirror. Are you benevolent toward yourself? Are you benevolent to your partner? Are you benevolent toward life?

Look even more deeply and ask: are you harming anyone or anything with your thoughts, words, and actions? Remember, benevolence is more than good intentions; it is kindness in action.

Now—gaze benevolently upon yourself, your partner, and the whole of life, especially any troubled circumstances that are crying out for healing. It is said that unhappy people are mean. Soften any hardness within, so you may look with the eyes of love upon everything—the morning rain as it washes your windows, the hooded eyes of a terrorist and his captives on the news, the sun rising like ribbons above your head, and your own face as you gaze into the mirror.

Many saints have said that prayer is simply receiving God's benevolent gaze and extending it out into the world. Look into your own eyes. Give and receive divine benevolence.

BIRTHING

Birthing—the action or process of giving birth to physical and non-physical creations

We are experiencing an awakening of the Mother Force upon the planet. You may have noticed that the word *birthing* is used much more these days, especially within creative and spiritual communities. But do we really know what it means and what it takes to truly embody this particular quality of the Mother?

A woman birthing an actual baby is a raw channel for the Mother Force. She is surrendered to the power of life itself as it moves through her. In this surrender there are moments of stillness as well as waves of intensity that she must ride. Inevitably there is a definite time to push her creation into the world. All of this requires *everything* she has and more, and it is made infinitely easier when she is balanced by her partner's total presence. These attributes of physical birth offer a metaphor for birthing all of our creative ideas. By embodying the feminine quality of birthing, we activate passion, we surrender to the power of the life force, and we fully give of ourselves, completely devoid of selfish ego. A woman in childbirth quickly discovers that she can't think her way out of this, and she can't make it painless—but the Mother Force in her will do *anything* to birth a safe, healthy baby. When she surrenders to that feminine power, she is a pure expression of Shakti.

Modern women do not always value the importance of having a strong connection to the Mother in their bodies. This particular manifestation of the feminine principle—both human and divine—makes us a channel for the life force. It will also open and expand our inherent sensitivity and deep feeling within the erogenous zones. Whether or not we give birth to children, maintaining our connection with the energy of birthing will enhance our creative activity. It will heighten our ability to radiate and passionately enjoy sexuality, ultimately revealing the precious jewel within—the mystery of rebirth.

The purpose of sexuality in the new paradigm is to open up the fullness of one another's hearts and to birth a divine creation together.

Mary Magdalene, the bringer of sexual holiness, knew that the ultimate stages of birthing the Divine Human were only possible with the balance between a devoted Frater Mysticus and Sororoa Mystica. This mystical brother or sister is someone intricately and karmically linked with you in a multitude of ways: someone who is your soul's beloved, heart's beloved, body's beloved, and fellow apostle in the depths of the great sacred work. Together this couple creates a mystical, tantric, and physical bond in order to fulfill their work on Earth. The man's mission in the world is nourished by the woman's feminine energy, her Shakti. Mary Magdalene, the embodiment of the feminine Christ, knew these mysteries well. She was instrumental in Yeshua's (Jesus's) mission. Her energy was different, but equal. Together they were in balance and their creation flourished for a time, until it became coopted by the patriarchy—and women's role in Yeshua's mission was written out of history. In order for the new paradigm to flourish, recovery of the original teachings is essential.

The mysteries of co-creation and birthing lie at the heart of the Magdalene's Path. By following her example, we can rediscover the essential elements of birthing so desperately needed at this time and birth our new Earth in balance, by activating our unique gifts and offering them to the world. All new creations are birthed from a harmonic balance of opposites—the union of masculine and feminine within—which results in balanced relationships in the world.

So how do we birth in balance? By women being women and men being men. By returning to our inherent natural template, without the dynamic of suppression and dominance. We would be wise to cultivate a simpler lifestyle that supports the different but equal roles of masculine and feminine. For most of us, both men and women, that will mean realigning with the feminine aspects of our being in a society dominated by patriarchal values. As women, we need to avoid being over pressurized and stimulated, multitasking, *always* putting others' needs first, and expecting that we can be *out there* and *in here* at the same time. We can consciously steer clear of any tasks or projects that stimulate our masculine tendencies. Men on the other hand, can open themselves to the importance of feminine wisdom and beingness. They can seek out the time for themselves to enjoy this quality of life—taking the time to rest, relax, play, and delight in and engage with the natural world. In essence . . . relax and let go.

Once we have we returned back to balance, the Mother energy within the woman will begin to flow and her natural instinct to create a family, a project, a home, a garden, and an offering to her wider community will flourish. In essence she will radiate, flower, and blossom into an unspeakable beauty that is both visible and felt. This will nourish the man immensely, and he will be inspired to support her creations with his own gifts. He will also have the energy and light for his particular mission in the world. As their balanced synergy expands, she will be brimming with offerings and the desire to give, circulate, and share all the talents within her.

In the past this abundant feminine energy of creation and birthing frightened the insecure masculine. Men saw that a woman could bleed and not die, that she had an innate power to not only bring forth life, but to sexually consume him and then wither his manhood. These primal fears triggered a shadow response to control the feminine and disallow her expressions. Yet ever since women were suppressed and considered mere property to control, masculine creation has run amok. Without the balance of feminine energy, man has spawned technologies of destruction—guns and weapons of all kinds, nuclear arms, drones, coal-burning power plants, chemical warfare—the list is endless. The result of this unbalanced creation is that humanity can destroy itself in a thousand and more ways, and Mother Earth herself is suffering. The Goddess always creates balance, however, and Earth is in the midst of a cataclysmic restoration of her balance, despite the cost to humanity.

As we know, much of the current imbalance is a response to the recent patriarchal phase of history. But keep in mind that the idea of God as purely masculine has existed in *less* than 5 percent of our history. Prior to this, humanity worshipped the Mother. Now the balance is again shifting, but in a new way that honors both men and women. In order to birth this new time, women must first acknowledge, and then completely release, any spiritual rage against the patriarchy that they may feel. This rage, whether conscious or unconscious, prevents women from returning to their true feminine expression. To serve this birth, men are invited to step forward and help women feel safe enough to express this rage, empowered enough to release it, and loved and accepted enough to move beyond it. The ecosystem and the entire Cosmos is sending out a call—it is imperative for men and women to wake up and birth the new paradigm together.

So, I ask:

Women: Are you at peace with your body? Do you delight in your yoni, womb, breasts, curvy softness, moistness, mouth, tongue, lips, and belly? Are you embodying your ability to nurture, love, let go, forgive, surrender, allow, be pregnant, make love, bleed with the moon, and welcome motherhood in all its forms and every primal aspect of the Mother?

Men: Are you able to awaken the Divine Feminine within yourself and balance it with your Divine Masculine? Are you willing to use this energy to empower your partner by assisting her back into her spiritual feminine self? Do you love the body of your partner, even if it is not perfect by the false standards set in the media? Can you help her feel her juiciness and innate sexuality? By loving her body and encouraging all aspects of her spiritual, emotional, and physical expression, can you help her to deeply awaken her feminine Shakti? Are you ready to fully empower a Goddess and be her divine equal?

Dearest friends, we stand upon a new threshold—a time of birthing through balance.

In the new paradigm, an awakened man celebrates the feminine birthing power as the Shakti that nurtures and strengthens him, filling him with life force for his own beautiful creations in the world. He encourages his woman to feel the Mother energy flowing within her. His natural creative energy loves to birth structure for her creations: he builds a home that she decorates; he tills the garden that she fills with flowers. She in turn warmly invites him to make love to her and worship her as an incarnation of the Goddess, thus restoring him to his rightful and divine role as a pillar of incorruptible light. Together they are the natural caretakers of Gaia and of all life.

This great rebirth—both planetary and within our human family—will lead to a sexual and relational opening in both genders. Because men and women have released and let go of shadow emotions, we will not walk in fear and we will not desire to control. Our offerings to the world will be just and true, and we will birth a new divine creation together.

Have you picked this wisdom key because you desire to birth something out into the world? Do you feel frustrated because you know there is more that you and your partner could be offering together? Do you feel a burning desire in your soul to come together in holy purpose, and to birth a new creation?

Well beloved one—you have picked this key for a reason. Here are some steps to actualize these deep inner feelings.

Holy Prayer

✦

Beloved Mother Father God, bless the coming of this new creation, which has a thirst not only for mother's milk, but also for the Source of the milk of life. Bless me [us] with bright eyes and a bright mind that discerns [bright minds that discern] the truth. Bless me [us] with a heart [hearts] big enough to see through the suffering of this world into the source of joy. Grace me [us] with hands that are creatively able to shape forms of love and feet that are grounded with strong roots, that do not forget where they have come from. Purify and clarify all my [our] intentions, blessing me [us] with a passion to serve life. Bless me [us], Mother and Father, with a new love that awakens the soul of this creation through the illusion of the world. Bless this sacred birthing space. Bless me [us] as protector and womb keeper. Help me [us] open into the intimate womb, that great vastness that all creations come from and return to. Amen.

⑤ Sacred Action

With your partner (or within your own being) birth something beautiful today—a mandala (a circular illustration representing the Universe in Hindu and Buddhist symbolism), a song, a poem, a dance, a blueprint for a building, a business plan to benefit humanity, a garden—the possibilities are endless! (Hint: Your holy purpose is engraved in your soul, and when you come into contact with a person that is willing and able to birth with you, you shall feel its predestined awakening.)

Ask yourself: When your gifts combine with your partners,' what is born? What is it that both of you would delight in sharing with the rest of your brothers and sisters? What breaks your heart in life? What are you deeply moved by? What creative energy within draws you to contribute to life?

Then work to manifest what you have discovered into your life. Remember that the movement from divine idea to physical manifestation is like an actual birth; it will have passion, times of slowdown, times of intensity, and a time to push! Trust the process and engage in it fully.

BLESSING

Blessing—divine favor and protection; the act of extending love and protection

I think God might be a little prejudiced.
For once He asked me to join Him on a walk through this
    world,
and we gazed into every heart on this earth,
and I noticed He lingered a bit longer
before any face that was weeping,

and before any eyes that were laughing.
And sometimes when we passed
a soul in worship God too would kneel down.
I have come to learn: God adores His creation.

SAINT FRANCIS OF ASSISI,
"GOD WOULD KNEEL DOWN"

No matter *what,* and no excuses, you must tell your partner how unbelievably gorgeous, beautiful, sensual, loving, delightful, radiant, strong, and desirable he or she is! Tell your beloved that it is a privilege to love him or her and how you desire to learn to love him or her more. We don't do this to feed his or her ego, but to create a harmonious field that blesses him or her. Giving and receiving blessings magnifies the divine in both of you.

I (Anaiya) find that this is similar to how I pray to God. God doesn't need me to love and glorify him-her, but in the actual act of worshipping and blessing in this way, *I* come away feeling expansive and sincerely more loving. It's the same with our partners. If we do not already do this and if we feel some resistance, we have to ask ourselves *why.* The gift of blessing expands our deep appreciation of one another and truly blesses all of creation.

The birth of the Divine Human is our next stage of evolution. In this phase we experience a unification of our highest and lowest natures alchemized together in our hearts and expressed in sacred action.

The birth of the Divine Human happens through the alchemical vessel of Sacred Relationship, both within yourself and in blessed union with your beloved: someone with whom you can fully give and receive love.

This tantra between emerging Christs is heightened and anchored during the act of love. Here, you find yourself passionately and openly blessing your partner and allowing him or her to bless you, so you can both be filled with the golden energy of divine passion. This is not something you do with the mind; you simply let go into the truth of your union and become enraptured by the grace of your meeting in the body at this precious moment in time.

Can you imagine telling the beloved for whom you have waited your entire life, *Excuse me, but I am not quite ready for this great blessing. Can you come back next week, next month, next year?* You don't turn the beloved away! All your life you have been waiting for this moment. How can you hesitate? How can you consider asking love and blessing to await your perceived readiness? How can we distance ourselves from the majesty of love that is *always* attempting to pour down onto us and up into us? But we do, don't we? We must be humble and ready to receive, Dearest Friends, for the timing of this invitation is not up to us.

And so, let us bless one another. Let us rain glory upon our partners and all of creation. Let us praise and worship one another's beauty, clarity, and willingness to step into the crucible with each other. Let us tell our beloveds what an honest and sincere job they are doing—even if our ego minds may judge otherwise. Judgment stops the flow of blessing and divine love. As we give, so shall we receive.

Holy Prayer

———————✦———————

Beloved Mother Father God, help me find within my heart the full capacity and sincerity to bless in your name. Open me to receive blessings—from you, from others, and from myself. Help me to not criticize or judge, but to rain down blessings, encouragement, recognition, and praise. Help me to create a harmonious field in which all can thrive and flourish. Beloved God, thank You from the bottom of my heart for orchestrating the meeting with my beloved. I bless You for Your help and for hearing all of my prayers. Let me never take my beloved for granted. Help me to love more unconditionally each day. Amen.

§ Sacred Action

Whom do you love the most? What ten people would you put on a lifeboat in case of a universal tsunami or an end-of-the-world scenario? Make a list.

You may have a million friends on Facebook, but at the end of the day, you are lucky if you can find ten people you would die for and who would die for you. E-mail or call them as soon as you can. Extend your love and blessings to them. Remind them that if the world ends tomorrow they will be on your lifeboat.

The truth is that we never know when our time is up. Humans can be the most forgetful creatures. We eat, sleep, and drink every day; let us also remember to love and bless.

♪ Additional Sacred Action

Spend this day silently blessing *everyone* you come in contact with.

Extend your love and light out to bless all beings and all of Nature.

Make it a habit to bless all things you see and use and all beings you contact—and watch how gratitude and joy grow! Now imagine the Divine Ones doing the very same to you, every day and night!

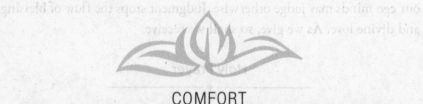

COMFORT

Comfort—a state of physical ease and freedom from pain; a person or thing that helps to alleviate difficulties

Comfort is a quality within the wisdom keys that is essential for the great rebirth. If we cannot comfort one another, we will not be able to cultivate a nervous system that can withstand the velocity of this intense alchemical process. We need to be calm, secure, centered—connected to *all* of ourselves and all of life. Yet in order to comfort another, we first need to feel comfort within ourselves.

Discomfort usually begins in the mind as a twisting and turning thoughtform that births an emotion, flooding the body with chemical messages that tell us to protect, run away, or disconnect. The next thing we know, we are in a fearful, divided, and separated state. When this happens, we have to remember that it all begins in the mind. And so we must eavesdrop on our thoughts—what are we thinking? Then on the heart—what are we feeling, what are we *really* feeling? Furthermore, no information of any significant value will arise unless we are breathing deeply and consciously.

Let us realize that the greatest, most loving, harmonious form of comfort is available to us anytime and is in abundance the moment we chose to activate and receive it.

There is a saying: *God is closer than your own breath.* Well what if the presence of God actually *is* our breath? In Hebrew, the word for spirit and breath is the same—*ruach.* The same can be said in Greek (*pneuma*). In fact, even in English the word *spirit* comes from the Latin word meaning breath—*spiritus.* When we look at the words *inspiration* and *respiration* (drawing in breath and the general process of breathing), we can see the connection, as they contain the same *spirit* root.

The soul is the inward, invisible part of us. The body is the outward, visible part of us. The spirit is the active life of the soul within the body. The soul requires a body in order to palpably communicate with others. Here in the body we have access to words, feeling, intonation, rhythm, and touch. In essence the soul *needs* the body to express and feel itself *fully.* Yet even with soul and body together, there is no communication if the body is mute and inactive, with the breath shut down. A body that is breathing and spiritually active can speak and communicate. The breath, or spirit, gives the body a voice, animating it. In fact, *anima* is the Latin root of the word *soul* in several Romance languages. So breathing *animates* our body, the vehicle for our soul. It allows our activities, words, thoughts, and feelings to be shared with others.

The Holy Spirit is often depicted as the Holy Sophia, the feminine aspect of the Godhead, and her presence bestows comfort and wisdom. Connection with the Holy Spirit births a comforting sensation of loving clarity that instantly reveals profound levels of wisdom. This divine energy heals, corrects, and harmonizes all involved. All it takes is some deep breathing. In times of uncertainty allow yourself to feel all your feelings, allow the body to become liquid, and stop trying to figure everything out with your mind. Then ask the following questions.

Holy Spirit, what is the truth of this situation?

Holy Spirit, what would you have me say, do, decide?

Holy Sophia, what within me is arising to be healed?

Holy Sophia, how may I assist you in healing and harmonizing my beloved?

Holy Spirit, what steps can I take to further prepare, heal, and deepen?

The Bible's Book of Wisdom is often attributed to the wise King Solomon, but it was actually authored by an unknown writer. It has many beautiful passages about Sophia. In chapter 7, verses 25–26, she is described as being "the breath of the power of God, a pure emanation of the glory of the Almighty, so nothing impure can find its way into her. For she is a reflection of eternal light, a spotless mirror of the working of God and an image of [God's] goodness."

So in this wisdom key we come face-to-face with the importance of breath. Your breath is the doorway to instant comfort, wisdom, and deep, deep counsel with the Holy Sophia herself. Let this never be forgotten—breath is the immediate gateway to God. It is the very process by which universal intelligence flows from God into the body itself, here and now.

Trauma in the womb, at birth, and during the early formative years, followed by cultural indoctrination that passes the tensions of our parents and ancestors into us, literally twists the free flow of breath right out of us. The health of our being at every level depends on how well we are breathing—and now you understand why.

I will close by sharing profound words taken from Jean-Yves Leloup's translation of the Gospel of Philip, verse 127, "If someone experiences Trust and Consciousness in the heart of embrace, they become a child of light." As you pray the following prayer and the Holy Spirit descends . . . pause with the internal dialogue. Fall back into the sensations—and *breathe*.

Holy Prayer

————————◆————————

Beloved Mother Father God, help me to let go. Help me to become still. Help me to connect with my breath. Help me to feel the Holy Spirit. Help me to open up a channel with the Holy Spirit. Beloved Holy Spirit, Beloved Holy Sophia, please come to me, comfort me, enliven my soul with your kindness and wisdom of life. Amen.

ৡ *Sacred Action*

Prepare a holy space where you will not be disturbed. Build a nest that is comfortable and warm. Play some soothing music in the background.

Come into a comfortable lying down position with your feet flopped open and your palms face up. If you are with your beloved, you could lie together on your backs as you gently hold hands or simply lie separately.

Close your eyes and allow your shoulders, neck, throat, jaw, and forehead to relax and let go.

After a good five to ten minutes of long, deep breathing, bend your knees, placing the souls of your feet down, and slow down your breath and heart rate by breathing in deeply through your nose. Then, hold your breath. When you are ready, slowly exhale through your mouth.

As you breathe in through the nose, feel how you are breathing in the Holy Spirit, along with the oxygen in the air. Feel the presence of Sophia, the Comforter. Know that the desire and necessity to breathe is God's divine spark of aliveness within you.

Feel that desire to breathe; connect with that desire to be alive; contemplate *aliveness*. What does this mean to you?

Then, as you hold your breath, expand your sense of the indwelling Holy Spirit: Sophia, the bringer of wisdom and comfort.

Finally, as you breathe out, feel all fear flowing away with the carbon dioxide, so that you can live freely in love, presence, and power. As the long exhale releases all forms of control, separation, and division, consciously offer all of your activities and agendas to the Holy Spirit to harmonize, correct, and comfort. As the comfort penetrates your being, you can also use your exhale as an oceanic wave that shares God's loving presence with all of life.

Breathe in. Hold. Then exhale and repeat.

§ *Additional Sacred Action*

With your beloved, massage one another's hands and feet.

Massage one another's head, neck, and shoulders.

Through this massage, learn how to relax the nervous system and stimulate the glandular system to secrete optimal levels of hormones. Help one another to stay in balance—and enjoy the deep sensual pleasure of massage, touch, and breathing.

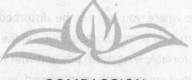

COMPASSION

Compassion—sympathetic concern for the sufferings or misfortunes of others

Compassion is not only the desire to ease the pain and suffering of another person or oneself, but also the *ability* to do so. To be able to serve the awakening and healing of another, you need to be able to look deeply into the heart of things as you contemplate the wisest, most far-reaching response. Shallow pity is not compassion. Compassion is robust and all-encompassing and is known throughout the world as being the essence of a *bodhisattva*—an enlightened being who has chosen to delay his or her own place in paradise in order to help others become free of suffering. One of the most well-known bodhisattvas is Kuan Yin, whose name means "regarder of the cries of the world."

One of the most touching stories of Kuan Yin tells of when she was disguised as a monk. As a young girl all she wanted was to study dharma and become a nun, but her father forbade her to do so and threatened the local nunnery against accepting her. Determined to live a spiritual life, Kuan Yin disguised herself as a young boy and entered the monastery to become a monk.

As the years passed she would often be seen outside tending to the gardens. A local woman became enamored by her and wondered how she might win this beautiful monk's attention. One day the woman became pregnant, though she was not married. In her despair and suffering she went to the head monk of the monastery and said it was Kuan Yin who had made her pregnant. Kuan Yin was immediately called in for questioning. When asked whether she was responsible, Kuan Yin—still disguised as a monk—said yes. In her great compassion she chose to forsake the spiritual life she loved so she could take care of the pregnant woman. By the time Kuan Yin died, her capacity to endure all indignities and her boundless spirit of enlightened service led her to paradise to become the Goddess of Mercy. Yet despite her prestigious title and guarantee of eternal peace, she still chooses to return to Earth again and again to help all those who are suffering and will continue to do so until all souls are enlightened and free.

Holy Prayer

✦

Beloved Mother Father God, help me to embody the greatest depths of compassion. Grant me the same openness of heart that Kuan Yin demonstrated. Help me to move beyond my limitations and the margins of love and kindness. Support me in extending Your great and all-embracing love to all. Allow me to rest in Your goodness, so compassion may flow from me unobstructed. Amen.

§ *Sacred Action*

This sacred action is a practice from the Tibetan Buddhism path of awakening. It is called Tonglen, which is Tibetan for "giving and taking." This sacred practice allows us to come into connection with suffering—both our own pain and the suffering all around us. It is a method for overcoming the fear of suffering and for dissolving tightness in the heart. Primarily, Tonglen is a method for awakening the compassion inherent in all of us, no matter how cruel or cold we might seem to be.

This practice is contraindicative to the human ego's way of seeing itself in the world. Truthfully this practice goes against the grain of wanting things on our own terms: wanting everything to work out for ourselves, no matter what happens to others. The practice dissolves the armor of self-protection that the mind creates in order to feel safe.

But it is important to remember that we are not taking this path of divinization, this path of radiant embodiment, merely for our own private liberation. Fully embodying this path allows us to be present in a devastating life experience with peace, courage, focus, and above all, boundless compassion, because *love* characterizes the essence of the Divine. As we do the work, we realize that we are here on the Earth readied and prepared to be used by God—in whatever way, in whatever difficult circumstances—to deliver the healing presence of the Divine Human, acting from within the sacred heart.

We have included this practice because we believe this sacred alchemy spurs us on to enter the final unconditional depths of our compassionate nature. Here we get to taste the deathless and undefeatable divine strength of love. Embodied in our sacred hearts, this love spreads its fiery energy throughout our whole being and makes us active flames of divine love.

The bodhisattva vow at the core of Mahayana Buddhism and the commitment of the Christ Path to total, radical, and joyful surrender both point to offering one's energies for the benefit of all sentient beings. Here we have the deepest imaginable truth of the divine embodiment process. This truth actively serves the awakening of all beings that are able to make that vow and sustain the necessary focus, commitment, and love in all circumstances.

So now let us turn to the practice itself. We're going to do it in three stages. In the first part we will be working with our own karmic, biographical self as we turn to face and clear the shadows and obstructions that cause our suffering. In the second part we will be working with someone we love who is going through a hard time physically and/or emotionally. The third part is where we turn our attention to someone who has caused us great suffering. Here we truly get to embody the great power of this practice as it shows us the real depths of compassion. When you practice Tonglen for those whom you are tempted to blame and shame and reject, not only do you help them on the inner levels, but you also work on the part of yourself that is like them. This sacred alchemy becomes a double divinization, which takes place at the subtlest levels. You cannot offer great depths of compassion to others unless you have truly partaken in it for yourself.

The Three Stages of Tonglen Work

Healing your own self

Healing the one you love

Healing the one who has harmed you

ꙮ Part One

Come into a cross-legged or standing position naked in front of a mirror, preferably a full-length mirror.

Stand or sit and look at yourself in the mirror. Know that the being who is looking into the mirror is your Christ self, your divine self—or whatever name you give it. This is your true essence: the one who has never been born and will never die. Know that your divine self has as its nature boundless peace and boundless passion united, boundless wisdom and boundless love united. Know that one of the most profound impulses of the divine self is to radiate selfless, all-transforming compassion. Know that the heart of the divine self is infinite, like the vast sky.

Know that the being reflected in the mirror—with the wrinkles, the sadness in the eyes, the lonely signs of pain and despair, the exhaustion, the weariness of life—is the karmic biographical being that is living and dying. Know that it is infinitely precious to the conscious divine being.

Gaze at yourself, from your divine self, with total lack of judgment at what you recognize: all kinds of sorrows, all kinds of fears, all kinds of fragilities, all kinds of vulnerabilities, all kinds of loneliness, and all thoughts, such as, *Oh my God, does the world have to be so dark and my path so difficult in this moment?*

Whatever arises, simply allow it all and keep witnessing with your divine self.

Now—imagine that all of these fears, doubts, and lonely emotions coming out of the belly of the being in the mirror in the form of a viscous ball of black smoke—very thick, very fierce, and extremely intense. Imagine that the divine self takes that black ball of smoke from your biographical self, absorbing it into his or her sacred heart, which is a vast, cloudless, radiant, sun-drenched sky. Clearly see the pure golden blue of that sky, and watch the ball of black smoke as it dissolves. Let all of that raving, black, viscous, tormented, nasty black smoke just disappear in the boundless sky of infinite compassion that is your true divine heart, your Christ or Buddha nature.

When the ball has completely dissolved, then from the full confidence of your divine heart, from the full faith of your divine peace, from the full passion of your divine compassion, radiate back to the being in the mirror all the joy of your realized nature, all the peace of your awakened nature, and all the compassion of your divine-love nature. Saturate that human self with radiant golden light emanating from You, to you.

Then speak whatever words come most naturally to you. It could be something like: *From my awakened heart, I radiate love, healing, power, hope, and divine energy to you. I take every obscuration, shadow, fear, and doubt from you. And I give you, with great love, the full glory and boundless blessings of the divine nature that I Am.*

You will find that this is a supremely powerful practice. When you come to dark places and savage disappointments in life, having this practice in your quiver will make the difference between falling into despair or trucking on with joy and faith and rugged hope.

❧ Part Two

Now we're going to do exactly the same practice with somebody that we know is having a very hard time at the moment. You are still sitting/standing in front of the mirror as you close your eyes and begin to imagine this person, with all of the pain and difficulty coming out of his or her belly toward the sunlit, pure, radiant, spacious sky of your divine heart.

Remain in love and openness. Absolutely know that you cannot be harmed by the pain coming toward you. Any voice inside that doubts this process *is not you,* but simply your own small-self fears. Lovingly set them aside and *be* the Divine Presence.

Fearlessly open the sky of your sacred heart. Watch the black smoke from your unfortunate suffering friend move into your heart. See it dissolve into nothing.

Stay connected to your divine nature as you radiate back to your friend all the healing, all the love, all the peace, and all the passion and compassion of your essential divine nature.

In whatever words are truly appropriate for the situation, speak your prayer to your friend. You may say something like: *From my awakened heart, I radiate love, healing, power, hope, and divine energy to you. I take every obscuration, shadow, fear, and doubt from you, and I pray that you receive, with great love, the full glory and the boundless blessings of the divine nature that lives in me.*

If you do this regularly for your friend, even without mentioning it, some change—some miraculous shift in the situation—will appear.

◆ Part Three

Now, we're going to turn to the grueling but gorgeous task of summoning up someone in our past—or perhaps in our present—that has done very radical harm to us, whether consciously or unconsciously. It is very powerful to do Tonglen for someone who has consciously caused you harm, because that is the hardest to forgive. I assure you that if you work with this practice, you will be able to overcome all initial resistance. As you commit to the inner presence of the Divine, you will eventually be able to tap into the depths of your compassion and bring forth a whole wellspring of unconditional love that forgives the one who once caused atrocious suffering.

With this third aspect of Tonglen, we taste the depths of the enlightened nature and how endlessly calm and brave it can be in any circumstance. It might inspire you to remember that the Dalai Lama does this very practice for the Chinese who invaded his homeland.

Still standing in front of the mirror, now, in your imagination, turn toward a person who has caused harm. The first one that comes into your heart and mind at this moment is probably the best person to do this exercise with.

Think for a moment of the woundedness or ignorance that may have caused his or her behavior. You may not know all the details, but imagine as best you can all the traumas, all the wretched decisions, all the cruelties, and all the destructive choices this person has experienced. See all of it condense into a viscous, black ball of smoke. Watch that black ball pour out of this person's stomach and invite it into the great spacious sky of your own radiant-heart nature, where it dissolves into thin air.

Pray that this person can be freed from whatever conglomeration of traumas, shadows, wounds, and ethical, moral, or spiritual decisions that led him or her to harm you. From within your sacred heart, you know that whatever others inflicted upon you, they inflicted upon themselves, because in the end, there is no separation.

As you dissolve that ball of black smoke in the core of your sacred heart, begin to radiate back thoughts of compassion and forgiveness. You may say something like: *I truly forgive you. I absolve you and forgive you. If I could, I would take the karmic consequences of what you did from you. I will pray that they can be taken. If they can't be, I pray that they will lead you deeper on the path of liberation. I pray that whatever has made you act in the ways that you have acted will be healed by this invisible practice that you may know nothing about, but which is given to you and to your soul's journey out of free will and love.*

As I said before, you may find this practice difficult at first, but please persevere. I promise you—grace comes to help.

DEVOTION

Devotion—love, loyalty, or enthusiasm for a person or activity

Aching

My Beloved, every wakeful moment with you is sacred. You
have burst the banks of my heart, so my love spills over.
This exquisite torrent is all that I have ever longed for since
the moment I was born. Your beauty warned me of this.
Your heart took mine to one side and whispered sweetly to my
devotion. Beware my love, for I shall break this heart. And
in this breaking you shall be free to love me with the depth
you have ached for.
I knew you would come, even as I crawled through the ashes
of your predecessors. I knew you existed and would one day
show your face again, inviting and receiving the sweet nectar
of my devotion. You have birthed new life in me, and your
lips are the holy cup my mouth begs to drink from.

Your heart is my inspiration and your soul my resting place. Your hands have caressed me into total surrender, my vulnerability leads the way to love you more, and the tears in my eyes reveal the truth of this overflowing commitment to love.

ANAIYA SOPHIA

The quality of devotion can spill from us in a passionate torrent of love. It can also be embodied in the quiet, daily repetition of the tasks required in caring for a beloved elder or child.

All of life is an altar upon which we place the offerings of our devotion. The practice of devotion pulls forth our best human qualities: generosity, passion, commitment, desire, patience, humility, surrender, joy, willingness, and unconditional love. Devotion opens us in ecstatic communion with the Divine and also fills us with gratitude for all the simple gifts of life. Devotion uplifts us to a higher octave; it is prayer in action.

Holy Prayer

✦

Beloved Mother Father God, help me reach into my devotion so I may feel the great depths of love You placed within me. Open me, Mother, so I may love with the whole of my body, and free me, Father, so I shall not fear its consequences. Glorious Soul, fill me with the trust that is Your inherent nature so this life is lived in devotion to God, embodied in word, action, and feeling. Amen.

☙ Sacred Action

Ask yourself: Where are you abandoning your devotion and opting instead to live a mundane life? What devotional acts can you embody today?

Devotion is the key that will unlock your heart and free your soul to love as you have longed to. Devotion is a feeling that flows out into action. Devotion needs an altar upon which to place its offerings—who and what shall be this altar?

Delight in acts of devotion. Let this sacred feminine quality shine through you today.

Read "Aching," the above poem of devotion, again, and invite yourself to become aroused and inspired by this transmission of love in action.

What words can *you* allow to course through your body and animate your pen? Allow preposterous words to irradiate your imagination and let them have their way with you! Allow the language of longing and love to spill out onto the page.

And then . . . read it to yourself and, perhaps, to your beloved.

ELEGANCE

Elegance—the quality of being graceful, refined, sovereign, dignified, and stylish in appearance or manner

The face is the soul of the body.
LUDWIG WITTGENSTEIN, *CULTURE AND VALUE*

We all recognize an elegant woman when we meet one. We can tell when we hear her speak; we notice her when she enters the room; we are comfortable with her integrity. She does not threaten, challenge, put down, or push forward. Elegance does not require permission, approval, or recognition from anything outside of itself. A woman's serenity, sincerity, and intelligence are all attributed to the inner elegance that radiates through her, imbuing the world with her charm.

An elegant being is one who is self/soul contained and whole in heartfelt beauty and refinement. This is immensely attractive to everyone. One does not need expensive clothes, makeup, or the latest sunglasses to be elegant. It comes from an inner bearing, a quality of radiance.

I think we could agree that Princess Grace of Monaco, Audrey Hepburn, Jackie Onassis, and Princess Diana are examples of women with true elegance. But what *exactly* is the quality that differentiates an elegant person from the rest? And more importantly, how would you birth a sense of elegance within you? What does it look like, and especially, what does it feel like? Where does it come from? What would you have to heal and release in order to embody it?

Elegance is a feminine expression, yet it is not limited to women. Men can also be elegant, incredibly so. Look at Steve McQueen, George Clooney, and Johnny Depp.

I understand elegance as a generous and all-inclusive expression of self-confidence. It includes the manner in which a person shines, charms, and brings others into their own radiance. Elegance carries an attentiveness and presence that lets other people know they matter and their existence is meaningful. An elegant person looks people in the eye when speaking to them, and gives them her full attention. Elegance never rushes anything; it acts as though it has all the time in the world—and so it does. Elegant people are centered, and they act as though every conversation they have is the most important one of the day. Elegance carries a certain warmth of heart, a palpable intelligence, and a conscious awareness characterized by simplicity and extreme clarity. Truly elegant people radiate contentedness, charisma, and authenticity, along with a sense of refinement that is both seen and heard.

Holy Prayer

✦

Beloved Mother Father God, I am willing to experience my elegance. I stand before You as pure emptiness. I want to embody Your warmth, charisma, authenticity, and contentedness. Provide the nourishment of Your beauty and grace now and every moment to me, as I seek only to refine and uplift. Help me release any distractions within and around me that may seek to dilute this pure intention. For You are the All, the Absolute and Only Being, of which I am born. And through You all shall become good, holy, and beautiful. Amen.

§ Sacred Action

Beloved Friend, you have picked this wisdom key for a particular reason. Ask yourself the following questions: Where are you calling for a sense of elegance to enter your life? Where have you been embodying or experiencing a sense of brashness? Do you feel any pushiness arising from insecurity?

Allow the palpable infusion of elegance to uplift your words, actions, and deeds.

Spend some time feeling into the more abrasive expressions within your life, and elegantly apply your charm and natural worthiness to their cry for attention.

If others do not respond to such a refined presence, then move your attention to a more noble cause. Elegant beings choose their company and environment wisely. Their nature is to uplift, not to be pulled down.

GRATITUDE

Gratitude—openhearted appreciation; thankfulness

A grateful heart naturally overflows into irrepressible joy—and joy is a telltale sign of the presence of the Divine. The practice of genuine gratitude opens the heart and fills it to overflowing. "My cup runneth over," wrote the psalmist. "Surely goodness and mercy shall follow me all the days of my life, and I shall dwell in the house of the Lord forever." Here the "house of the Lord" is a metaphor for living in a state of Divine Presence and pure gratitude. Brother David Steindl-Rast, an Austrian Benedictine monk, is a Christian contemplative with a deep understanding of Eastern spirituality. He calls gratitude "the heart of prayer." Gratitude leads us naturally to mindful awareness and it opens our hearts to the mystery of Presence, an awareness of the Divine in all things. He says, "if we call it mindfulness or wholehearted living, it is easier to recognize prayer as an attitude that should characterize all our activities. The more we come alive and awake, the more everything we do becomes prayer."* Gratitude can cut through our perpetually dissatisfied ego and quickly lift us up into the energy of prayer, praise, and thanksgiving.

The more we abundantly practice gratitude, the more things we will

---

*From Brother David Steindl-Rast's *Gratefulness, The Heart of Prayer: An Approach to Life in Fullness* (New York: Paulist Press, 1984), 48.

find to be grateful about! Gratitude is like a small, potent seed; whatever we are grateful for will increase multifold in our lives. By consciously choosing to plant this seed in our minds and hearts, huge blessings will unfold. Gratitude is an attractor of energy—a powerful alchemical tool to be used daily. It is amazing that simply making a gratitude list can quickly lift one out of a bad mood. Positive people tend to gravitate naturally to gratitude, always seeing the cup half full; pessimists often perceive by focusing on lack and judgment, even if their lives are filled with everyday blessings. People who have come through dark tragedy and who can still see the bounty of life are those who know the secret of happiness—a grateful heart.

For, in truth, when we can wrest an attitude of gratitude even from difficult circumstances, we quickly turn negativity around and also penetrate to the heart of whatever spiritual lesson we need to learn. I remember when my late husband and I totaled our car. Waiting for the tow truck, we stood on the side of the road in January, *freezing*, and numbly saying, "We are so grateful to be alive! And somehow, this is for the highest good!" It turned out that since the accident wasn't our fault, the settlement we received was generous enough to help us build our dream house in the mountains.

Years later, when my husband died of cancer, I really prayed to find the good in it, especially for my children. I kept telling them to trust that there was a gift hiding in that awful time. Now, as young adults, my children have a deep connection with the invisible world, which they forged by seeking contact with their father and finding that his presence was still available to them whenever they needed it. It has served them well, and they are grateful for their deeper connection to the Mystery. They trust that things happen for a reason and that a lesson or gift is *always* there to be found. This attitude can bring us into automatic alignment with the Divine and keep our hearts open, even through pain and difficulty.

Author and self-help teacher Louise Hay reminds us to bless our bills as we pay them; to fill our hearts with gratitude for the services received. What a blessing! Taking this attitude in life will magically ensure that we have plenty of money to pay the bills and more, especially if we give thanks in advance. Thich Nhat Hanh has a beautiful practice of giving thanks to every organ in the body by greeting it with a smile and sending it love and gratitude. Try it, and see how your body responds with health and joy. Expressing our thanks to the people who serve us coffee, pick up our garbage, take our tickets, or pack our groceries at the store is a way to share gratitude with others. We may never know it, but this simple act of extending love could change someone's life. So, my dear friend, please remember that *every* aspect of life is truly magical when lived in gratitude!

Gratitude is an essential tool for Sacred Relationship, especially when partners get caught in judgment or wounding. Gratitude helps us to step back from the small picture, which we so often use to illustrate a big story in our mind. It can unlock the ego's grip and put us back into a heart-centered space with our partner. The truth is, our big story of wrong and right is usually an ego fabrication. Ask yourself, *Would I rather be right or happy?* If we are willing to get off our high horse, most of us would really rather be happy. When we take a moment to breathe and express our underlying gratitude for all the blessings our partner brings to our life, our hearts will open into love. From that place, it is easy to use our communication skills to work out an issue.

Appreciation is an expression of gratitude that really nourishes sacred union. It is a wonderful practice to find something each day to appreciate about our partner and to share it aloud. No matter how long you have been together, make a conscious effort to *never* take your partner for granted. He or she is a living divine mystery, ever changing and alive. Cultivate this attitude, and activate gratitude for each other in new and creative ways! Remember, too, that expressing gratitude for all the things we love about our partner will magnify those things. Women especially flourish when their partners praise what they want to see more of, rather than criticize what they don't like. Yet *all* of us bloom and expand in an atmosphere of gratitude and appreciation. It is supremely important to consciously fill our relationships with that energy.

Gratitude expands the heart into a huge conduit for love. It is the energy that draws all good into one's life. It is the gateway to joy and the companion of true humility. Gratitude keeps us aligned with the present moment and helps us to remember what is truly important—love.

Holy Prayer

---✦---

Beloved Mother Father God, thank You, thank You, thank You! This human incarnation is a huge gift and blessing. Thank You for everything you have so lovingly sent my way—I know it has all served my growth. Thank You for my body, this amazing vehicle I use daily without much thought. Thank You! Help me to take nothing for granted. Thank You for this beautiful Earth that nourishes and sustains me—Mother Gaia, help me offer grateful service to you. Beloved Divine, help my heart to stretch even bigger in gratitude and joy! Expand my capacity to love and to be thankful for everything—the "good" and the "bad"! I am so grateful for [name everything and everyone you are personally grateful for in your precious life]. Amen.

◎ Sacred Action

Make a gratitude list right now.

Every day for the next month, add one new thing that you are grateful for. This practice will help you to be mindful as you live each day and discover new reasons for gratitude—large and small.

As you lie in bed each night, share what you are grateful for with your partner or with yourself.

When you wake in the morning, let your first thought be one of gratitude for your cozy bed and your night of sleep. Then open your heart to the bright new day filled with opportunities to extend love and feel gratitude.

Give thanks in advance for all that you desire to be and create, and watch miracles unfold!

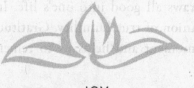

JOY

Joy—a feeling of great pleasure and happiness bubbling up from within

The transfiguration of a relationship is birthed by the powers of joy, revelation, ecstasy, adoration, honesty, and suffering in authentic mystical growth. Without all of these qualities being present and embodied in balance, divine alchemy cannot take root. Every single ingredient is essential. Here it is, right here—the divine mix.

It can seem as if both joy and sorrow run parallel to each other in our lives. As Khalil Gibran shares in *The Prophet*, "The deeper that sorrow carves into your being, the more joy you can contain."

When you're in the midst of an amazing experience, do you have a nagging realization that maybe it's not perfect? And when you're experiencing something painful, do you also get a sense of the glorious realization that there is still beauty and loveliness to be found? At the beginning of the journey toward divinization, it may seem as if these two qualities flip-flop. Ultimately you will take that magnificent leap of faith and enter the readiness to experience the unbridled and wild fullness as joy arises, bringing all sorrow to the forefront of your consciousness to be felt, embraced, and released into yet more joy.

How did we find joy? By saying "Yes!" to God.

Divine joy bubbles up for no external reason or purpose. It is the very current, fabric, and substrata of creation and the basis of the Divine Human. Divine joy is part of God's love, and is inseparable from it. It is the very infallible sign of Divine Presence! Joy lives in you *as* you—and it increases as you shift from living in the ego-mind to living in the heart.

Wonder, an aspect of joy, is a childlike emotion. Wonder arises when something new and singular is presented and memory cannot dredge up any image from its archives that resembles this strange encounter. The body responds by shamelessly staring, opening the eyes wide, suspending the breath, and swelling the heart. It is such a delightful feeling!

These bodily symptoms point to three dimensions that are essential components of wonder. The first is *sensory:* wondrous things engage our senses—we stare and widen our eyes, ears, nose, tongue, and touch. The second is *cognitive:* such things are perplexing to the mind as we cannot rely on past experience to comprehend them. This can lead to a suspension of breath akin to the paralyzed response that kicks in when we are startled: we gasp and say, "Whoa!" Finally wonder has a dimension that is spiritual: we look upward toward God, divine intervention, or a miracle in veneration, hence the swelling heart.

Wonder means you do not know. It brings a fresh and open appreciation of yourself and your partner. It makes all things new. Wonder makes us little children again, open to rediscovering ourselves, others, and the world in a new way. Wonder cleans our mental slate, making our minds a blank canvas to allow our hearts to bloom. Wonder opens us up to new experiences and elicits joy. Isn't this worth it?

Wonder, joy, innocence—they are all the same thing.

So beloved, are you willing to look on and be present with your life in joy and wonder? Let go of the old-paradigm mind with its incessant need to know and open to the beauty and innocence of having no fixed answer! Joyful innocence has no judgment, no preconceived idea of what anything or anybody is—including you. Let go of figuring out or thinking you know someone else, or even yourself. Anything is possible. Why not open to this and see what happens? This makes life more fun and more filled with joy!

In India it is said that God created the Universe for no other purpose than to simply express joy and delight. Why? . . . Why not? The answer is joy. We are the expression of God's joy and delight. This is how we have been created. This is who we are. Christ shares that only creations that bring more love into the world have any value. Joy is part of love, as love is part of joy.

Holy Prayer

✦
___

Beloved Mother Father God, please pour Your divine love into me.
Open me to joy! I welcome joy into my being, as I release my defenses
against joy. Beloved God, You are the one birthing me, bringing to
my door every single circumstance for me to open up to. I throw my
arms around You and all Your ways of awakening me. I offer You no
resistance in this moment. I am open. I am ready. And I am desiring
all of You. Show me joy, God, fill me with ripples and waves of ecstatic,
mad, wild happiness—along with the quiet and deep eternal faith
that you are reeling me in to allow me to live in the presence of joy
forevermore. Amen.

Sacred Action

Do something that brings divine joy. Take a walk in Nature and listen to the joy of the birds, feel the joy of the sun, the joy of the earth beneath your feet. Feel the joyous kiss of the rain and the joy of a falling leaf. Feel Nature in your heart and know with certainty that the Universe is vibrating with joy.

Now—say "Yes!" to your life, *all* of it. Recognize that the feeling of joy arises when you fully trust that God is the orchestrating force that births and brings into wholeness all the details, circumstances, and beings that enter your life. Hold to the deep trust that ultimately *everything* is all right. Make a determined choice to praise and thank God in every situation. Joy and wonder can spontaneously appear when you know that every ring of fear is *not* God or someone doing this *to* you, but rather, God or someone doing this *for* you.

Look at the areas in your life where you are experiencing sorrow, rough edges, friction, and growing pains.

Now look at them through the lens of understanding that God is doing this *for* you in order for you to become more of your true, joyous self.

Breathe long, slow, and deep breaths as this realization fills your being.

Allow the breath to soften what could be rigid within as you open, relax, and surrender in this moment to the absolute truth—God is doing all this *for* you. Let all the mental junk that keeps you bound in sorrow, or in a victimized stance, just wash away. God is doing all this *for* you! How crazy and wonderful! It is all really okay!

Laugh. Let joy arise. You are loved beyond measure. Joy is your birthright!

Beloved, drop into your breathing before asking the questions below. Allow yourself to simply witness or become aware of the answers that appear, much like an innocent child would simply observe, without editing, judgment, or analysis.

What is the most significant sentence for me in this Pearl of Wisdom? What does it mean for me? Is there any sentence in the reading of which I find my breath changes or emotion arises? Resistance? My mind begins to race? Is there any part of me that doubts, wavers on, questions, or minimizes this Pearl of Wisdom?

Am I willing to truly allow my entire existence to be full of wonder and joy? What shift can I make in myself that would allow this Pearl of Wisdom—and the import of its acceptance—to settle more firmly into my bones during the next two weeks? How might that shift show up in my daily life?

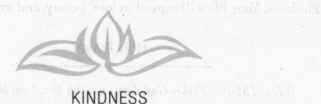

KINDNESS

Kindness—the quality of being friendly, generous, caring, empathic, and considerate

You cannot do a kindness too soon, for you never know how soon it will be too late.

RALPH WALDO EMERSON

Before you were born you knew that there would come a moment in time when the course of your life changed as you discovered the divine compass within you. You knew that in the process of your return from separation to oneness, you would choose to hold back your divine gifts so you could fully learn the worldly reality that you were birthed into and understand its rules and conditions. You knew you would temporarily forget many of your gifts. You did this to fit in and play the game of separation. You chose this of your free will, knowing that one day, you would awake, and your divine compass would change direction without hesitation, compunction, or delay. You knew you would call forth your inner gifts and detach from the world of greed and control. You knew you would turn inward at the perfect moment and say "Yes!" to God. Beloved, the moment is here; it is now!

All it takes is a shift in perception from fear to love.

Everyone around you is here to help you to love more, no matter how he or she is acting.

You have one duty—to love, which is to be in constant union with the Divine. One of the most beautiful expressions of love, or unity, is kindness. True kindness to oneself and others imbues our aura with a steady golden glow. Because we realize our oneness with all creation, we naturally treat others the way we would like to be treated. Use your divine compass to look for opportunities to practice random acts of kindness. Your life will expand in love, beauty, and joy.

Holy Prayer

✦

Beloved Mother Father God, I am one with You. I am love manifested. So be it. Amen. [Repeat three times.]

§ Sacred Action

Beloved Friend, let go and breathe into your heart.

Connect with the feeling of kindness, for you are only surrendering to your own essence. Remember there are only two expressions of love: one is a clear extension of love; the other is a call for love, maybe disguised under the pretense of anger, sadness, or conflict. When we encounter these negative feelings in another, through the kindness of our hearts we will never take offense or take things personally.

Now take yourself back to a moment of conflict, fear, or anger with another. Can you feel, underneath the tension and argument, that it was really a call for love? Feel this now.

Feel the energy of your soul guiding you, holding space for you. Ask your soul to increase its presence so that you can feel *its* love and kindness. And then relax . . .

Allow your soul to pour out its gratitude and kindness for *you*, for all your efforts and growing pains as you continue to endure and experience the soul's birth into the manifested world. Breathe.

Please pay no attention to the doubters—either within you or outside of you. Even if you encounter naysaying, snickers, and sneers—that is none of your business.

Love is your business. You—the one who reads these words—*you* are kindness. Let it shine, Beloved, let it well up inside of you. Let it pour through every cell of your aura and heart as you fill with kindness and extend love more and more every day.

> *My religion is kindness.*
> THE DALAI LAMA

MOTHER*

Mother—a woman in relation to a child or to the creative expressions to which she has given birth

In many cultures within the old paradigm, becoming a mother was seen as an obstacle to becoming a Divine Human. Parents simply did not have the time and energy needed to meditate for hours every day, as was the norm for the path of enlightenment in many traditions in the past. This reflected a profound separation between human life and the Divine. However, motherhood offers the opportunity to merge both.

---

*This pearl, which is mainly directed toward women, is parallel to the Father pearl (page 118), which is mainly directed toward men. Of course everyone can gain from reading and absorbing the importance of both pearls for the masculine and feminine essences inside all of us.

This capacity to merge the two is built into our physiology and soul as a direct means for our soul embodiment here on Earth.

The moment a child is born, the mother is also born.

OSHO

Innate within motherhood is the sustaining nurturance and stillness that we need in order to live in our multidimensional self. There becomes less separation between meditation/prayer and life, because all life becomes an authentic opportunity for *being love*. Being love is the ultimate catalyst for soul growth. In every experience that arrives at a mother's doorstep, she is offered an opportunity to choose love, whether it may be self-love or giving and receiving love with another.

Many cultures believe a woman is not a full woman until she has biologically and soulfully bloomed through the portal of birth into motherhood. The permanent changes in a woman's body and brain in this process stimulate the magnetic circuitry of her feminine self. This brings her into an innate receptivity and an infinite capacity for giving—directly from her body and soul to those she loves. Selfishness dies, and vast amounts of patience are born in this extension of love called motherhood.

From this loving heart-womb space we have the capacity to make whole, nurture, tend to, and love others. To live in *mother essence* means that we align *with* and navigate *from* our heart-womb space. When we don't, it is a sure sign that an emotion is arising that needs to be felt and released.

The foundation of family love is fertile ground to unlock some of the deeper recesses of the feminine soul. We must be connected intimately to our partners, ourselves, and God and have a continual flow of giving and receiving love to sustain us.

"Ma" is one of the most commonly used words among all languages. When we step into Motherhood, we activate the energy of "Ma." We step into a deep, vast river flowing with the ancient lineage of mothers. We become one from whom sustenance flows. This flow of life force is a flow of love. It physically moves through us in the process of birthing, and then as milk from our breasts. This life force energetically moves through us as love. In this great flow, we become part of the fractal web of life.

Motherhood opens us deeply to the tenderness of all life, the precious vulnerability in ourselves and in others. Embodying the Mother also awakens us to a fierce protective instinct. The Mother embraces everything that life brings in one moment—and in the next moment, she lets it all go. Motherhood is the continual process of birthing something from our most intimate place within, and releasing it out into the world in love.

Motherhood is an initiation into a deeper aspect of the feminine soul. It is a call to be birthed into the next octave of our being. It asks that we listen with our purest intuition to the flow unfolding through us and around us. This flow is continually birthing the next step of our evolutionary expression, of our souls, our relationships, our projects, our prayers. Motherhood fortifies our trust in God. It is here that we receive guidance for everyone's best interests, and it is here that we receive our soul's next unfolding.

Motherhood is an invitation to deepen into one of the purest and wisest expressions of the feminine. Motherhood is the marriage of intuition, wisdom, awareness, and love with action and manifestation, here and now. The journey of being a mother is not about leaving all things human behind in our search for God. The journey is about surrendering to the experience of being human and finding God through this.

This awakens a true compassion. This compassion is fuel to enact our earthly purpose, what moves us to bring heaven to Earth, to uplift the old paradigm into the new paradigm. This is Shekinah, the feminine principle of God-in-action working through us on Earth, fully embodied. This is how a mother becomes the Divine Human and helps birth the new paradigm.

Holy Prayer

———————✦———————

Beloved Mother Father God, please help me become the true mother within me. Spark this remembrance within me! Help me feel and release my pain, sadness, lack of trust, and hurt with my own mother.

Beloved Mother God, I know You are always here for me. Help me be here for my partner and children—and myself. Amen.

⑥ *Sacred Action*

Connect to your breath and ask yourself these questions: Do you feel the need to control your partner at times? Do you trust your intuition? Do you feel unresolved anger or frustration with your mother? Do you provide yourself with all that you need? Do you take time to process your emotions? Do you feel resistance to your partner's emotions? Where does your guidance come from? Can you express the truth even if it is hard for others to hear? Do you have clear boundaries in your relationships? Do you withhold love from anyone? Are you honest with yourself and your partner?

Then connect to your breath again as you ask yourself these questions concerning your own mother: Did your mother try to control your father? Did your mother trust her intuition? Did your mother provide all that you needed? Did your mother nurture you and freely give you love? Did your mother abandon you? Did your mother show and process all her emotions? Did your mother show resistance to other's emotions? Did your mother express the truth? Did your mother have strong boundaries? Was your mother comfortable in her own body? Did your mother enjoy sexuality? Did your mother enjoy motherhood? Was your mother honest?

When you have answered these questions, simply bring awareness to what came up. Breathe deeply, witness, and allow.

NATURE

Nature—the phenomena of the physical world and all its collective forces, including the elements, plants, animals, landscape, and other features and products of the Earth

Mother Nature, or Gaia, is an important part of our design for union and birthing the Divine Human. Connecting to her electromagnetic flow allows us to deepen into our own electromagnetic flow. Mother Nature is the beginning and end of the human journey—where we start on the path and where we realize our union. It is the alpha and the omega.

Only when you have fully connected to Nature and walked through this doorway can you fully connect to all other realms. Nature is the gateway. Being fully grounded, being soul-spirit connected to your body, is the gateway to God for the Divine Human. Nature is where the physical and spiritual meet. It is where we are born and how we are reborn.

Nature does not exist in isolation from us or from the rest of the Universe. It is a living part of our Divine Human blueprint. Earth Mother, the Spirit of Gaia, and Divine Mother, are all part of one wave. They are not separate, as we have been led to believe. In this union is the solid ground for the birth of the Divine Human. This is the queendom where the actions of God on Earth happen. *It feels like love in action.*

It is vital to connect to Nature every day, to ground yourself into your true blueprint. The action of the Divine happens on Earth. In India there is a saying: "God's work is done by God's servants, humans on Earth." God needs us to do this work here. We need Earth to be our support; we need to give to the Earth so it can also blossom as well.

The Divine Human living on the fifth dimensional Earth is being birthed. What that looks like, no one knows, because it has never happened before, but it will happen. It involves merging the physical body with the spirit body and the soul.

Gaia helps us with this by conducting and relaying information between different forms of life through DNA. There is a higher magnetic power latent within your DNA. Such magnetic power is the foundation for the Law of Attraction. Until you resonate with the Earth's hum, the grace of this law is not fully realized in your life, your path, your embodiment, or your relationships. Earth is the attractor.

Nature grounds us and aligns our desire for union. Whenever your frequency is out of alignment with Gaia's frequency, you are out of alignment with your natural rhythms—genetically, spiritually, and physically. As Earth's fields are now changing rapidly, so too does this frequency, and this is the cause for many of the disturbances in us, and on Earth, today.

Many of our deepest charged memories, emotional identities, and emotional reference points—both positive and negative—are held within the Earth's magnetic fields. As we open to the web of life, the web of interconnection, the web of Gaia, we access more of these memories. As you feel the emotions held here, you can welcome aspects of your soul back into the here and now. In feeling them and being present with them, they are released. This frees the soul to be present in the moment.

As proof of the power of Nature's magnetic fields, NASA astronauts found that when they first left the Earth's orbit and magnetic fields, they went slightly mad because they lost connection to some of their memories and identity. NASA learned from this, and now every astronaut has a magnetic attenuation box on his or her belt.

Holy Prayer

✦

Beloved Mother Father God, ancient presence of this land, I open myself to You and the mysteries of Your natural world. Open me, Mother, so I may absorb Your presence through the supportive powers and principalities of the invisible worlds. Help me come in to feeling communion with You, as the embodied Godhead, here on Earth in everything that I see, hear, taste, touch, and smell. May the core of my being fuse together with Yours as I come to realize, once and for all, how the joy of union is here. As I rest within You, may all the components of my body be restored, recalibrated, and suffused with Your living breath.

৬ Sacred Action

Feel the space within you that knows and feels Mother Earth. See and feel, in your heart's eyes, a beautiful place in Nature that is your sacred site and power spot, the place in Nature you *most* resonate with: a river, a park, a forest, a sacred site, wherever comes to you immediately. See the details: the beach, the ocean, the trees, the animals, the birds, and all the different kinds of flora that are in your special power spot. Feel this place. Open to the elementals, the fairies, the invisible ones that govern the cycles and flows of nature's harmony.

Let yourself begin to feel the love, the gratitude, the appreciation that you have for Mother Earth. Keep deepening this experience of love, repeating, *I love you, I love you!* until it gets to the point where you can feel this throughout you.

Once you feel this begin to open your root, at the base of your spine, as you send your loving essence with your intention to feel nature's response directly down to the center of the Earth.

And then just wait for Mother Earth to send her love back to you. When you feel this love coming back from the Mother, for she will *always* give you her love because *you are her child,* let it move throughout your heart, your soul, your body, *through all that you are.* Hold back no secret place from this love.

In this moment you are now connected with the Mother in love. You can stay here for as long as you wish, feeling this love, absorbing her wisdom, appreciating this connection.

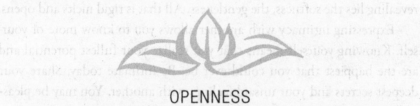

OPENNESS

Openness—the quality of being freely available and accessible to share one's thoughts or feelings

Openness requires vulnerability, transparency, and total honesty. When these emotional and soulful actions are integrated within you in daily life and in all your relationships, then you enter the quality of openness.

Total honesty requires that you share what you feel and think, even if you are concerned your partner may not like it! This does not mean being rude, arrogant, or unkind. It means being honest and not concealing your real emotions from your partner. Taking responsibility for these emotions and thoughts and sharing them in a gentle, open way allows real dialogue and exploration to occur.

When you express something, you also release it. Just through expressing yourself about touchy topics, the energy unfolds and can resolve gracefully. The pent up energy of anxiety, stress, and worry can unwind and release, enabling you to feel unburdened, clear, and free.

> *My grace is sufficient for you, for my power is made perfect in weakness.*
>
> 2 CORINTHIANS, 12:9

Expression is the medium for transparency. Without expression there is no intimacy. Our willingness to express and be transparent brings a beautiful vulnerability—love's naked openness. Transparency is the pathway for the new consciousness. One only enters this path by openly expressing.

Deeper expression allows you to be known. Becoming known means there are no more secrets, no more places to hide or retreat to. In the revealing lies the softness, the gentleness. All that is rigid melts and opens.

Expressing intimacy with another allows you to know more of yourself. Knowing yourself means that you realize your fullest potential and are the happiest that you could ever be. Be intimate today. Share your deepest secrets and your unsaid feelings with another. You may be pleasantly surprised.

This expression leads to weakening of the ego and keenly felt human vulnerability, which sublimely transforms as you openly allow yourself to be known by your partner and God. Your openness lets them both into every nook and cranny of your body and soul—willingly, humbly, and gratefully.

Vulnerability is part of humility. Vulnerability invites all of the secret places in our heart to come out into the light: all we are scared of, all we are ashamed of, and all that we hide in dark places within. Whenever you are openly vulnerable, your partner will feel it. He or she will be drawn to you, to comfort, hug, and hold you. It is a great attractor and inspires support. Vulnerability brings us all closer together and opens the way for someone to be at your side. When we are not vulnerable, we push others away and stop ourselves from receiving what we truly want: love. Vulnerability brings us the loving balm that our souls need to grow, and when we have integrated this into our daily lives with transparency and honesty, we become open.

Openness means we are open to whatever life brings us, knowing that it is for our good. Openness is the end of attachment to any outcome. We may still have preferences, but we are not attached to them. Openness is true flow, where we become like water, able to flow into any situation and environment. We can be speaking to a beggar one moment and a king the next, and we are equally open with them both, meeting them where they are, sharing what is needed to be shared in the moment.

Openness has no dogma, creed, or religion, no special jargon or language. Your openness resonates and speaks to everyone wherever they are. In true openness you won't lose your center or pretend to be something or someone you are not. It brings us directly and perfectly into the flow of life, the flow of synchronicity, the flow of the Law of Attraction. Openness allows us to share everything we feel without self-judgment, blame, self-punishment, or unworthiness.

Openness is a blank canvas that has infinite possibilities and infinite choices, none of which are good or bad. There is no dualtiy in openness—everything is seen as equal. What is good for you one moment may be bad for you the next; what is not appropriate for you today may be the best thing in your life tomorrow.

True openness comes from knowing your soul, because the soul is free and open. In openness there is emotional intelligence, strength, and softness, which come from having integrated transparency, vulnerability, and honesty. You access all these qualities in any moment, and there is no negativity, shame, or worry about it. Openness is a consolidation of all these qualities that brings a strong, fluid center, a core within you that is supple and powerful—yet open to change as well.

Having this foundation of openness means we are open to the greatest transformations. We can flow with whatever comes, secure and safe in our emotional center. We are open to the greatest alchemy of all—enlightenment—and we can accept it each moment as it comes. Openness brings us all we ever wanted, as we can now receive without barrier or block. God always wants to bring us everything. Can you be open enough to receive?

Holy Prayer

✦

Beloved Mother Father God, please help me open myself to Your love and Your will. Please help me open myself to my deeper emotions, hidden away inside me. Please help me open myself to all that life wants to give me, teach me, and share with me. Please help me open myself more to my partner. Help me be more vulnerable, honest, and willing to share all that is within me. Amen.

♪ Sacred Action

Beloved One, is there something you are not sharing? Is there something within you that you are concealing, about yourself, your partner, or your life?

Take this moment to breathe deeply and come into feeling communion with the deepest aspects of your true self. Allow the hidden to be revealed, allow the half truth to become full truth, become open, available, and accessible to your full and whole self.

Tell your partner three things you have never told him or her before. Maybe you did not tell your partner out of fear, out of being polite, or because you were ashamed to say it. Try it today. Be kind and caring. What happens?

PASSION

Passion—an intense desire or enthusiasm for something

Sacred Relationship is born through the unity of passion and peace.

ANDREW HARVEY FROM THE
TELESEMINAR *BECOMING A DIVINE HUMAN*

The birth of a new love-force is pouring down upon us. This golden energy is the great supreme gift of the sacred heart of Mother-Father

God. *This* is the gateway into the new paradigm. This love-force is the vibration needed for humanity's ongoing evolution. We believe this power is divine love awakening a new blueprint in our cells. A new kind of human being is emerging; we are becoming love's body, radiating in intimate communion with all that lives.

The key to fully utilizing this thrilling and often challenging time is to show up as love in action. Find something that is above and beyond you, something that you truly wish to serve, and pour out your gifts in service. The people I know in this world who are happiest are not those who are rich and powerful. They are people who have made the decision to live creatively as Divine Humans: fully alight with their unique soul mission and walking their talk in daily action. Those who show up like this are given nothing less than the wine of the Divine Beloved— an elixir of ecstasy, meaning, and joy.

The five great sacred passions below help us explore "how on earth" to live in this way.

Five Great Sacred Passions

1. The passion for the Divine Father, the great shimmering Creator of the Cosmos

2. The passion for the Divine Mother, the great adoring abundance, the manifestation of the One

3. The passion to fall in love with all living beings and experience an unbearable compassion for all sentient life as well as the whole of the natural world

4. The passion to love someone with your whole mind, body, heart, sexuality, and soul

5. The passion to put *all* of these passions into action and to serve the birth of the Divine Human

Holy Prayer
---✦---

Beloved Mother Father God, help me to become a midwife, lover, and sacred warrior of the way forward. Help me to be brave in the face of immense challenge, when my soul asks me to step forward into action.

Help me to not enter this path for my own sake, but on behalf of all of life. Help me to become luminous, brave, strong, passionate, wise, energetic, exuberant, and gutsy enough to pour myself out in sacred passion, especially in pivotal moments of tremendous growth. Help me to realize that, should I fall, I only fall back into You. Help me to live my life on purpose with a passion that shines like a thousand suns. Amen.

☙ Sacred Action

Take a look at the five great sacred passions above.

First feel into the depths of your being to sense how you inwardly respond. Feel what arouses you.

Then write down how you act on each one or how you could act on each one.

How can you align yourself with these passions? Have you selected this pearl because you are experiencing deadness in your passions? Have you fallen out of balance and sacrificed your purpose? Does your relationship serve these passions? Write down all your answers.

Allow yourself to unwind and unfold. Energetically align yourself with your passions and allow God to take care of the rest.

QUEEN*

Queen—the female ruler of a sovereign state, one who inherits her position by (re)birth

As this process of divinization takes shape and form within your own being all the falseness of the old paradigm will begin to fall away. Feelings of unworthiness, being unable to say "No," settling for second

---

*This pearl, which is mainly directed toward women, is parallel to the King pearl (page 143), which is mainly directed toward men. Of course everyone can gain from reading and absorbing the importance of both pearls for the masculine and feminine essences inside all of us.

best, ignoring or denying unconscious behavior (in self or another) will become uncomfortable and impossible to endure. This is a sign that the Queen is birthing within you. For this quality to anchor deeply it would be wise for you to midwife this gift of awakening by taking on the characteristics of the Queen and applying them every day.

In the old paradigm there were certain women who were naturally born to be queens. There was something about them, in their personality and how they spoke, which made it effortless for other people to admire, respect, and follow them. Now, *all* women being birthed into the new paradigm are being prompted by the evolutionary force within their own souls to learn how to develop and embody queenly qualities.

One of the first steps in becoming a queen is to understand how to harness your gifts and use them in the right way. While there is no set list of things that make a woman a great Queen, there are certain traits that an impressive, noble Queen *does* have. The first trait is authentic leadership by example. A true Queen's feminine power of love, as well as her graciousness and generosity, inspire others to emulate and follow her. The second queenly trait is complete willingness to accept responsibility. A Queen is willing to accept responsibility for the errors that she may make, and she deals with the consequences effectively. And the third important trait is this: when a decision needs to be made, she will decide and act, even if the decision is a difficult one. The Queen clearly understands her role as a ruler. When she has made her decision, she stands by it with a powerful, magnetic presence. Her radiance encourages others to love her and follow her.

Holy Prayer

✦

Beloved Mother Father God, You created me to be a Queen. I am one who intends to embody all the qualities of the Divine Feminine. I am ready to accept my responsibilities and claim the gifts and attributes You have placed within my own soul. I am willing to lead my life in the direction of my sovereign soul and to make the decisions that reflect and uphold my nobility. I am steadfast in my desire and I pray for Your internal promptings and grace. Thank You, Beloved God,

*for cultivating within me the ability to know and feel my worth, my
value, and my virtue. I and my Mother are one. I and my Father are
one. Together we are Creation. Amen.*

✍ Sacred Action

Beloved One, take some time now to breathe and embody the Queen
that you are rightfully becoming. Here is a breathing practice that allows
you to feel all the aspects of your feminine essence, as you become a
flow of magnetic light and breath, united and whole within yourself.
The more you are centered in this, the more you will feel *yourself*. This
exercise is especially beneficial to practice before making love, as then
all parts of you will be engaged, receptive, juicy, and open. This beautiful weaving between upper and lower areas of the feminine body allows
a deeper, grounded opening.

Inhale glowing, iridescent, deep wine red energy deep down into the seed of
your ovaries, the light generators of your body and fuel for your womb. Your
ovaries become glowing, iridescent, deep wine red with each breath. Do this
six times.

Now breathe this energy into the magnetic field of your nipples,
connecting them in a loop to your ovaries. Connect them with your breath
six times.

Breathe this energy down into your yoni lips, the entrance to the sacred
space of your womb and divinized sexuality. Connect them with your breath
six times.

Breathe this energy into your chin chakra, seat of your queenly authority.
Connect it six times with your breath.

Breathe this energy into your gratitude g-spot inside your yoni. Connect it
with your breath six times.

Breathe this into your womb, the grail, the center of your power, and the
foundation of your heart. Connect it with your breath six times.

Breathe this into your sacred heart with love. Connect the heart energy
with your loving breath six times.

Breathe this into your pineal gland, your center of vision and illumination.
Connect this stream of vision and illumination with your breath six times.

SEXUALITY

Sexuality—the capacity for sexual feelings and experiences

For a woman to open up to her immense natural sexual fullness, she must trust a man with her whole heart, soul, and sacred feminine core. As women, we need to feel that our partner recognizes us as an incarnate form of the Goddess. In turn men need to recognize that their masculine energy is deeply nourished by the sensual feminine. Furthermore, through bold and fearless surrender to this holy feminine Shakti force, a man can embody the full power of light at his sacred masculine core.

Woman's Sexuality Work

As women, we are 100 percent responsible for opening and releasing any blocks that prevent us from accessing our sensual feeling body. First, however, we have to recognize how the patriarchal age may have taken its toll on us.

In modern-day society, particularly since the 1980s, women have entered the workplace and been exposed to an incessant barrage of competitive power seeking. A new myth arose, which declared absolute gender *sameness,* and it quickly became culturally accepted. Part of this served to rectify an imbalance; women had certainly been subjugated and considered inferior to men in the past. But the balance tipped too far, and many women erroneously believed they had to behave exactly like men.

Many women have overanimated their masculine energy in the race for success and the drive to get ahead in their careers. Men and women alike have been culturally caught in the craving for bigger and better *things,* which creates anxiety around money and even more drive for worldly success. Eventually this leads to collapse and burnout—*especially* in women who have subverted their natural feminine energy.

Women with a strong feminine essence are not designed to be like men, yet for the last thirty to forty years many have pushed themselves in that direction. We women are not created to be out there in the world conquering, achieving, amassing, and owning. We are designed to be out there in the world creating, visioning, beautifying, nurturing, and balancing. The modern myth of gender sameness and society's overvaluing of masculine qualities has resulted in women being energetically located in their heads, disconnected from their sensual, sexual selves and primarily running on their masculine energy.

This is not good news for society or for the bedroom! Because we women have activated too much of our masculine energy, often out of necessity, we are unable to relax and trust men in the act of love. This problem is compounded because many men's innate masculine sense of direction and sexual empowerment has wilted in the presence of an overly masculinized woman who can't surrender to their loving. And equally problematic is many other men's misaligned use of masculine power based on society equating power with power over.

What I have noticed over the years, especially within the spiritual communities, is how the women seem to express their sexuality in a masculine way, and how the men in response have begun to express their sexuality in a feminine way. The ladies have become strong and initiating while the men have become passive and receptive. This is not sexy! That is why it is so important to address this disharmony between the genders. I believe we are reading this book because we recognize this and we want balance. We have reached a place where we are willing and able to connect with our masculine and feminine expression as and when it is needed and appropriate.

Another area that must be addressed is the widespread use of pornography. This issue is growing and seeping into society from as early as six years old. Many men in general are hiding this aspect of themselves from the container of Sacred Relationship, and it is not only causing a schism within them, but also in the deepening field of relating. If you want deepening intimacy, quite simply pornography has to go! It is designed to keep us in a state of separation, feeding an industry and intelligence that thrives on isolation and addiction.

It doesn't matter how many sexual skills we know or how open we are emotionally. If we women don't trust our lover's masculine expression and direction *more* than our own, we won't open completely. We won't let down our boundaries and surrender in deep trust, allowing ourselves to be sexually overcome by the Divine Masculine. And if we are stuck in our heads, there is a very good chance our masculine energy will not only match his, but also surpass it.

Now, there is another urgent issue for women to address. We must give ourselves permission to reawaken our feminine essence and heal our overly strong expression of masculine energy. Go deep inside and ask yourself if you can let go of all that conditioning and awaken the inner Goddess . . .

This may be more difficult than it seems, because staying in control has often kept you safe. But is a woman who truly desires sexual ravishment really interested in merely "staying safe"? Are you willing to take a risk for feminine bliss? If the idea of trusting a man is too much, simply begin by trusting life. Surrender into the flow of life that has brought you to this moment.

We can begin to awaken our feminine sexuality by going into Nature and feeling the pulse of the Goddess. Soak in a natural hot spring and feel her force bubble up between your toes. Sit on the Earth and draw her energy up through your yoni into your body. Go outside in a private place under a full moon, take off your clothes, feel the breeze on your skin—and *dance!* All these things—and many more—will awaken the sleeping sacred feminine within.

In terms of sexuality, we must also ask: do we know how to give *ourselves* pleasure? So many women are judgmental *of* and uncomfortable *in* their bodies, which can turn lovemaking into a painstaking chore, rather than an exploration into bliss. For us to fully access our sensual sexuality, we must quiet the mental voice that is constantly evaluating the sexual experience; otherwise we are still in our masculine energy. In the words of poet Mary Oliver, we must relax and "let the soft animal of your body love what it loves." For us to surrender into deep sexual expression, we need to be grounded in our being, rising from the Earth in pure delight as fully feminine women.

In summary here are the two important points for women to remember.

- A woman's lover's masculine consciousness, presence, and direction must be capable of bringing her to a deeper, more blissful, and abundant love than she is capable of directing herself to, or she won't trust him.
- Women must be capable of reconnecting to their sensual body, opening up to the womb, remembering the qualities and attributes of being female. They must allow their core feminine essence to swell up and rebalance their masculine energy, or their beloved will sense the over-masculinized energy within them and lose his instinctual interest.

Man's Sexuality Work

Men must learn to be ever more courageous in the face of limitations, remaining present and pushing through fear into the brilliant light on the other side. A primal masculine terror exists as well, which says, *If I really channel my divine heart light into the sacred feminine essence of my beloved, I may become completely consumed and overwhelmed. Her natural sexual fullness and inexhaustible ability to love may swallow me whole, and I may not even exist or be able to do something important ever again.* The greatest fear for the masculine is that the energy of Divine Feminine could consume him—so much so, that he would abandon the external drive that anchors his "importance"—status, money, career, reputation, and dominion over the Earth. What awakened men can realize, before it's too late, is that this very act of being consumed and swallowed whole is the portal to a complete *rebirth*. Moving through this fear and penetrating his partner with total focus will birth them both into light and ever deepening love.

Therefore, if a man really wants to open sexually as the Divine Masculine, he will not get to experience the deepest bliss of the sacred sexual feminine unless he is with a lover who can surrender more deeply than he can. With every fiber of his being, he also must desire to enter the sexual dance with the feminine. He has to be in touch with a wild longing to serve and merge with the Goddess, knowing that she is the absolute and only being that sustains him, creates him, and will one day dissolve him. As David Deida has eloquently reminded us in nearly all of his books, the awakened man's fearlessness in the face of this realization will propel him to love all life and ravish his woman with tireless strength and clarity. He looks directly at death and remains in the present moment while making love—knowing the part of him that is a man and the part of him that is light.

Once we have balanced our inner masculine and feminine, once we have developed as an autonomous, whole person, then we have achieved psychological integration. But to experience divine sexual bliss, there is another step to take, that of surrendering to the other's essence. It doesn't mean that we lose our capacity for wholeness in everyday life, but the masculine and feminine essences play entirely different roles in the bedroom.

Women—you can learn to relinquish your boundaries during sex, giving yourself entirely to be taken by the divine masculine force. And remember, if you want to experience the fullest divine play as the feminine sexual partner, then you must choose a lover worthy of your trust.

Men—you can choose to move through primal fear and learn techniques to control orgasm, so you can endlessly ravish your partner. Cultivate your divine masculine essence so that you attract a partner with a strong feminine essence and the willingness to surrender to your loving.

If your current relationship needs work in these areas, it doesn't necessarily mean that you must end the relationship and seek elsewhere. Love conquers all—so just look inward together and discuss whether this refinement of energy and technique is possible and if it is something that you are both committed to. As the man works on his ability to extend his whole-body depth of fearless presence, the woman can cultivate her capacity to receive his heart-true navigation. Just make sure, if you take the path of cohealing, that you follow up all conversations, insights, and agreements with an action step as soon as possible. Practice, practice, practice. It can be fun!

I have been speaking primarily to people with either a strong masculine essence or a strong feminine essence. These types, gay or straight, long to awaken the gifts of sexual love. But there are also people with a more neutral sexual essence, for whom the play of masculine and feminine is less important.

Ultimately love is what we all desire. You can enjoy love with your friends, children, and parents. You can love yourself. You can love the Divine. You can love your intimate partner in many ways—cuddling, gardening, or raising a family together. Love is the very nature of your being, the very nature of all Being. Love is the openness of every moment.

Yet . . . if you find yourself yearning for a love that *includes* ravishing sexual play, our prayer for you is that the words of wisdom in this chapter may help you along the path. Though we have outlined no specific techniques, no sexual tricks or erotic prose, we have offered an energetic map and a template. It's all about being able to embody these masculine and feminine forms of energy. Specifically, we are being asked to navigate and experience these forms of energy in a new, pure way. If we agree to these expressions within us, then we have the map of the Great Birth in our hands—the birth from the human to the Divine.

The way you make love is the way God will be with you.

RUMI, "BREADMAKING"

Holy Prayer
✦

Beloved Mother Father God, please help me [us] to become free
of all sexual conditioning, all sexual guilt and shame, all sexual
unworthiness and suppression. Help me [us] to throw off my [our]
sexual repressions, dullness, and deadness—help me [us] awaken
into the blissful ravishment of Your divine caress. I [We] know You
hunger for my [our] awakening into sexual bliss, for You planted
that gift in my [our] body [bodies]. Let me [us] be courageous

enough to say "Yes" to You and "Yes" to my [our] soul[s] by crying out a primordial "Yes!" to life. A life that is wild and free, tousled and galloping. Let me [us] not be afraid of entering the arena of surrender and ravishment, of being rocketed into Your majestic heart through the ecstasies of Your mind-blowing presence. You are my [our] beloved, and I [we] want You so much more than I am [we are] capable of saying. Amen.

☙ Sacred Action

Beloved One, let us delve into a sexual self-inquiry for you and for your partner. Take time, delve into each level of inquiry on your own and with your partner, and feel fully complete with each before moving on to the next. Feel free to breathe into and meditate on your answers or to journal about them. If you are not currently in relationship, simply keep the questions aimed at yourself and answer wherever possible.

Initial Inquiry

- Do I feel that I am/my partner is empowered?
- Do I feel that my/my partner's Shakti is flowing?
- Is my partner sexually compatible with me?
- Is my partner's sexual power stimulating for me or a turn off?
- Have I/has my partner done any self work on sexual healing?
- Is my/my partner's sexual energy connected to the heart?
- Do I really enjoy our lovemaking and does it fulfill all parts of me?
- Does my sexuality make me feel like a real woman or a real man?
- Do I feel loved and met in lovemaking?

Higher-Level Inquiry

- Am I/is my partner full of life, alive, and free?
- Do I/does my partner have a true and real center?
- Am I/is my partner grounded in self without need for anyone or anything else?
- Am I/is my partner able to make decisions clearly and effectively?
- Am I/is my partner free to do whatever I/he or she want(s)?
- Are my partner and I living the life we want to, or do we have excuses around that?

- Do I/does my partner have self-discipline, focus, and willpower?
- Do I/does my partner achieve things, or just talk about them?

The Shadow

- Have I/has my partner done his or her shadow work?
- Am I/is my partner integrated with his or her shadow?
- Do I/does my partner have the depth and substance that comes from having looked deeply within and feeling one's own darkness?
- Can my partner see his or her own shadow and my own?
- Is my partner willing to transparently talk about this with me?
- Is my partner willing to go into both of our shadows together as a couple?
- Do I/does my partner have a lot of unresolved mother-father issues and/or a lot of emotional baggage? And if so, is it worth being with my partner to support him or her through this, or will it be too much for me and for what I desire in a relationship?
- Am I/is my partner integrated and self-aware?
- Am I/is my partner in denial of the shadow side and/or unwilling to deal with it?
- Does my partner project onto me?
- Does my partner need me to be the mother or father figure, even unconsciously?
- Do I trust my partner enough to fully let go?
- Can my partner objectively reflect aspects of my own shadow back to me for my own growth?
- Am I/is my partner willing to be deeply, vulnerably human and weak?
- Does my partner deny, justify, and rationalize his or her life and actions?
- Is my partner frequently defensive?
- Does my partner refuse to grow and take actions for self-improvement and healing, despite what I share with him or her?
- Does my partner listen to me?
- Does my partner have a lot of expectations of me?
- Is my partner mature and able to reflect, self inquire, and contemplate well?

Boundaries and Balance

- Do I have to initiate most movements in the relationship?
- Do I have healthy boundaries? Does my partner?
- Do I have my own free space and time?
- Am I able to speak and be with my partner and truly communicate, even when pain is arising or shortly afterward?
- Do I love myself and maintain my sovereign center within the relationship?
- Do I often sacrifice myself for the other to maintain the relationship and keep everyone happy?

Sacred Relationship

- Do I feel that my partner is in touch with divine will, and if so, does my partner follow it?
- Does my partner follow a higher love and truth?
- Is my partner's own self the only reference and orientation point in his or her life?
- Is this person in touch with living wisdom and divine truth?
- Is this person genuinely receiving divine love?
- Is this person serving others, or just self-serving?
- Does this person have a direct, living relationship and communion with God?
- Does my partner just believe in God without the daily experience of the soul of God?
- Does this person believe he or she is God?

And exhale . . . Very insightful stuff.

Of course this self-inquiry also highlights the areas within *your own self* where love and awareness have not yet entered and where you seek wholeness outside yourself. So even doing this self-inquiry *by* yourself, *for* yourself, can be very valuable.

SURRENDER

Surrender—relinquishing resistance and allowing higher guidance, influence, or emotion to empower you

Most of us have been wounded in love at one time or another. I can understand why women sometimes hold back their love from men and don't surrender their hearts and bodies wide open to them. When this happens, we must ask: Why did we choose this man if we really don't trust him? What attracts women to men who fail to allow us to surrender and open in love without the tension of mistrust? And do men fail to open women into blissful surrender because they are also wounded and mistrusting? Perhaps this mutual mistrust is an unconscious residue of tension from the past. If so, it is our responsibility as conscious men and women to unwind this tension, and become truly ready for the deep surrender of love.

My Dearest Friends—there is a threshold we simply *have* to cross in order to reach this state of surrender.

Your lover is with you for the sake of love. He wants you to receive his masculine love, and he wants to receive your feminine love. She wants you to receive her feminine love, and she wants to receive your masculine love. He wants *you* to trust his gift of heart direction more than your own. She wants *him* to value her gift of heart radiance more than his own. Therein lies the heart of surrender. For the birth of a Divine Human, individual parts of the self must be offered to the crucible of love. In crossing this threshold, we cannot hold on to full autonomy.

A woman's true power is in her ability to surrender, for it is in the surrendering that a woman is able to fully receive. Surrender and receptivity often get mixed up with being passive, and that is where many women may see it as a weakness.

In this letting go to the other, you allow a man to worship your body's glowing beauty and your heart's light of divine love. He allows you to acknowledge and surrender to his heart's capacity to spiritually and sexually open you to God. This two-bodied devotion only works when two bodies are better than one: when, as David Deida says, "you are opened more by his deep command and heart-guidance than by your own efforts, and he is opened more by being drawn into your heart of devotion more deeply than his self-enclosure would otherwise allow him."*

If this devotional surrender is blocked, your independence and lack of surrender will evoke his independence: he will find ways to receive feminine radiance without you. He will spend time in Nature's radiance—surfing, hiking, and skiing—or he'll choose to relax with the energy of music or a soothing beer rather than with your unsurrendered heart. As a woman, if you are with a man who can't guide your body and heart open to God, maybe you are better at opening *yourself* than he is at opening you. If so, you are right in trusting your self-guidance more than his. But the question is—how much longer can this relationship last? You may have come to mistrust external masculine guidance—perhaps you inherited such mistrust from your experience with your parents or past intimate betrayal—and so you have chosen a man who justifies your fearful need to direct your own life. But this does not lead to the birth of the Divine Human. This does not invite love's fullness to flow unimpeded.

This does not allow either of you to surrender into Sacred Relationship. Your partner will feel your lack of trust, and you will feel the weakness of his loving command in your life. You can love each other as two independent and self-responsible people, but you will never surrender open in love's most blissful dissolution, and he will never commit himself completely in his claim of your heart. You would do better to stay in the safe relationship of two self-reliant and autonomous people.

But this book is about the birth of Divine Humans—men and women inflamed by the surge of love to go beyond a safe relationship.

Women—be willing to clear your inner wounds and then open to the frequency of a man that you *know*, deep in your sacred womb, is

---

*From David Deida's *Dear Lover: A Woman's Guide to Men, Sex, and Love's Deepest Bliss* (Boulder, Colo.: Sounds True, 2005), 113.

capable of directing and guiding you to God. Trust his ability to melt you into surrender.

Men—be willing to clear your inner wounds and then open to the frequency of a radiant woman who can surrender to your trustworthy direction and heart's love. Trust her radiance and love to open you beyond your fears.

Choose to say "Yes" with every fiber of your being to this Sacred Relationship, for it is a path to the birth of the Divine Human and a new paradigm for this Earth.

As you become ready to live a love larger than one body, remember that you always attract what you put out. A woman who worships a man's depth of masculine consciousness attracts and inspires a man who worships her heart of devotional feminine radiance. The openness you induce in one another through this worship expands your capacity to love far beyond each of your bodies, beyond even your two-bodied ecstasy, unfolding your love outward to infinity, connected in compassion to all sentient beings, even to the moon and sun and stars. Your sexual embrace can open you to God through the loving worship of masculine consciousness and feminine radiance.

Holy Prayer
✦

Women—*Beloved Mother Father God, please help me to surrender. Help me to relinquish the guiding control of my internal masculine. Help me to soften unto this man and allow him to guide me deeper and deeper into You.*

Men—*Beloved Mother Father God, help me to be a clear and pure channel of Your penetrating light, so I may cleanly and effortlessly guide this woman back into Your loving embrace. Help me to be an ambassador of Your divine truth and abundant love.*

Together—*Beloved Mother Father God, help us both to trust this process and to surrender deeper and deeper in love. Help us to surrender the small self and listen to the Holy Spirit, which is whispering constantly of our highest aspirations. Amen.*

§ *Sacred Action*
Practice the "Sacred Embrace" (below).

ALCHEMICAL BODY PRACTICE

SACRED EMBRACE

. . . and the holy of holies is the bridal chamber, or communion.
Trust and consciousness in the embrace are exalted above all.

THE GOSPEL OF PHILIP AS TRANSLATED
BY JEAN-YVES LELOUP

The Gospel of Philip is best known for its portrayal of the physical relationship shared by Jesus and his most beloved disciple, Mary Magdalene. Philip's gospel was suppressed and eventually lost until it was rediscovered at Nag Hammadi in Egypt in 1945 as part of what is now known as the Nag Hammadi library, a collection of mostly gnostic writings from the third century CE. What emerges through Jean-Yves Leloup's translation is a restoration of the divine union between the male and female principles that was once at the heart of Christianity's sacred mystery.

While reading the gospel, I (Anaiya) asked to receive the hidden wisdom within these teachings and the understanding of how this mystery can be reenacted here and now in this day and age. The sacred embrace practices that follow are what I received.

Summary of the Stages of Sacred Embrace

Sacred embrace within the self: the marriage between the masculine and feminine qualities within your body and soul

Sacred embrace with your partner: the marriage of trust and consciousness between the two of you, throughout all aspects of being

Sacred embrace with God: the marriage of human and divine qualities within your body, soul, feminine, masculine, self, other, and with God

◊ The First Sacred Embrace

Within every embrace, both internal and external, trust and consciousness must be expressed. This is the primary mystical key that births the two into one. Trust is the feminine aspect of the embrace and consciousness is the masculine aspect; when we bring the two together we resemble God.

Play some emotive music that invokes feelings of love and expansion as you bring the masculine and feminine together into a harmonious marriage of deep feeling and companionship on the inside.

Whether you are doing this practice alone or with you partner, come into a comfortable cross-legged position with a straight spine.

Close your eyes and begin to tune in to your internal masculine and feminine energies. Feminine energy in both males and females is situated on the left hand side, and the masculine energy is on the right. Your feminine energy is represented by qualities of love, kindness, patience, creativity, playfulness, joy, dancing, sexuality, nurturing, eating, comfort, and blessings. Your masculine energy is represented by qualities of truth, clarity, guidance, direction, decision making, choice, justice, protection, faith, discipline, and strength.

As you sit with your eyes closed, begin to connect with these two energies within you. As different qualities arise, recognize, acknowledge, and honor the sacredness of each expression.

Feel the two aspects embrace and accept one another.

At times this inner work may feel restrictive or confusing—just breathe and pray, as any resistance you may feel has simply come up for healing. When we first embark on our sacred union journey, we may feel distrust of our inner feminine or masculine. Internally, we may resist the idea of marriage between the two. Don't let these feelings put you off; they are quite normal. The internal world is most often projected out onto the external world, so the harmony between the masculine and feminine first has to be restored within.

Witness any resistance and continue to breathe deeply, taking the breath all the way down into the heart, torso, and sexual organs, allowing yourself to soften, to trust, to open, and to heal.

You may experience the rising up of emotions that may be both pleasurable and painful. Remember they arise to be healed—just continue allowing, trusting, and embracing these sensations so you may retrieve all the lost, forgotten fragments of your being. All is well beloved; this is the healing that the Sacred Marriage brings.

When you feel that you have come into a true and loving sacred embrace on the inside, move into the second embrace.

§ The Second Sacred Embrace

Now open your eyes and come closer to your partner, to include him or her in the sacred embrace. You are about to reflect outwardly what has happened on the inside. You may sit on top of your partner's crossed legs, in a pose known as the *yab-yum* position (see page 68) or lie down together and hold one another (see page 69). If you are practicing alone, you simply do the same thing in your imagination, choosing to sit or lie down in a sacred embrace.

Begin to extend the trust and consciousness that you are feeling inside to include your partner.

Again, at first there may be a few thoughts and feelings that arise to suggest that you can't or shouldn't do this. As we know by now, this is our cue to breathe deeper and pray to move beyond these wounded parts of ourselves. They have been incarcerated by the ego to separate us from sacred union. They judge and hold on to past grievances only out of fear. Get big enough to hold it all. Let go and allow love to be fully present.

As you come together, let both partners begin to feel each other's presence. Feel the breath, the heartbeat, the body, the energy, the pure love and consciousness extending toward you.

Imagine that this person is simply *more* of your self. Know the truth, that there is no separation. Invite yourself to experience how this second body is simply more of your own body; this added warmth, breath, and movement— both energetic and physical—is just more of your own self.

Utilize the breath to relax deeply in order to facilitate an experience of oneness and wholeness.

Extend love to your partner with all of your body, heart, and soul. Let no place within you be left out, despite its wounds and resistances. Love, trust, allow, heal, bless, and comfort one another. Trust his masculine energy; trust her feminine energy. Be conscious of his masculine presence; be conscious of her feminine presence. Trust your self; be conscious of your self. Trust the embrace; be conscious of the embrace. Trust the inner world; be conscious of the outer world. Trust the outer world; be conscious of the inner world. You see the alchemy that is forming here.

Now, take it further, into the third embrace—what more can you trust and be fully conscious of?

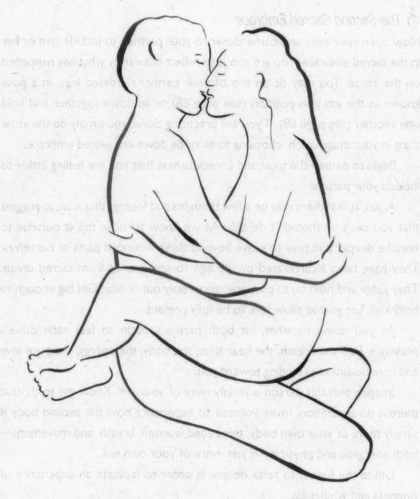

Sacred embrace in yab-yum position

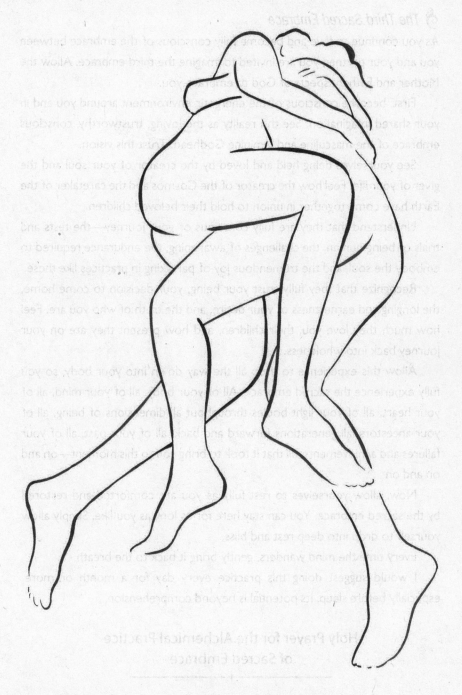

Sacred embrace lying down

ॐ *The Third Sacred Embrace*

As you continue to love and become fully conscious of the embrace between you and your partner, you are invited to imagine the third embrace. Allow the Mother and Father aspects of God to embrace you.

First, become conscious of the energetic environment around you and in your shared imagination. See this reality as the loving, trustworthy, conscious embrace of the masculine and feminine Godhead. Trust this vision.

See yourselves being held and loved by the creator of your soul and the giver of your life. Feel how the creator of the Cosmos and the caretaker of the Earth have come together in union to hold their beloved children.

Understand that they are fully conscious of your journey—the tests and trials of being human, the challenges of awakening, the endurance required to embody the soul, and the tremendous joy of partaking in practices like these.

Recognize that they fully trust your being, your decision to come home, the longing and earnestness of your desire, and the truth of who you are. Feel how much they love you, their children, and how present they are on your journey back into wholeness.

Allow this experience to drop all the way down into your body, so you fully experience the sacred embrace. All of your body, all of your mind, all of your heart, all of your light bodies throughout all dimensions of being, all of your ancestors, all generations forward and back, all of your past, all of your failures and achievements, *all* that it took to bring you to this moment—on and on and on . . .

Now, allow yourselves to rest fully as you are comforted and restored by the sacred embrace. You can stay here for as long as you like. Simply allow yourself to drop into deep rest and bliss.

Every time the mind wanders, gently bring it back to the breath.

I would suggest doing this practice every day for a month or more, especially before sleep. Its potential is beyond comprehension.

Holy Prayer for the Alchemical Practice of Sacred Embrace

———————————✦———————————

Beloved Mother Father God, Creator of our souls, help me [us] to trust fully, help me [us] to become fully conscious of Your presence working through my life [our lives] at all times, in all ways. Help me [us] to soften my [our] hardness, so I [we] may be able to fully love, to fully trust, and to richly partake in life. Help me [us] to tell the truth always, to others and myself [ourselves]. Help me [us] to become truly humble, so that I [we] let go of all my [our] attempts to be right or to be perfect. Guide me [us] into becoming vulnerable, soft, and kind-hearted. Help me [us], Mother Father God, to release my past [our pasts] with grace and forgiveness. Help me [us] realize that all I [we] have experienced has been orchestrated by You, and by my own soul [our own souls], in order that I [we] may grow closer to You, closer to love, and closer to truth.

Please imbue me [us] with the faith and strength required to partake in this holy union, both within myself and with my partner [ourselves as individuals and with each other]. Grant me [us] the perseverance to continue on when my ego [our egos] says to run, hide, or withhold. Grant me [us] gentleness of speech when my [our] wounds arise, grant me [us] patience for the work, and please, God, grant me [us] the maturity to not do what I [we] have always done in the past—but instead to rise up and to dig deeper into the rich soil of my true self [our true selves], to become noble, worthy, and grateful for all that You are patiently, relentlessly, and joyfully giving me [us].

> *In the Name of the Father*
> *And of the Sun (both son and daughter)*
> *And of the Holy Spirit (Mother)*
> *Amen.*

✦✦✦

Realize in this moment there is nothing else outside of this embrace, only the extending of the soul's expression as love throughout the whole of Creation. Allow yourself to experience this as you softly come to terms with these words from the Gospel of Philip: "That they shall resemble God . . ."

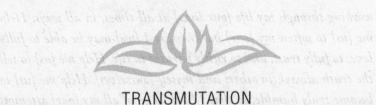

TRANSMUTATION

Transmutation—the action of changing or the state of being changed into another form

Fuse the powers of the sacred heart with the energies of the body, and you can transform everything.

PIERRE TEILHARD DE CHARDIN

Love does not die, nor does it end. Our relationships may come and go, but love carries on, free of our changes. Within the blueprint of Sacred Relationship there is a wealth of latent potential that can consciously transmute every form of disharmony, friction, and suffering. The masculine brings forth his steadfastness and diligence, while the feminine connects to her empathy and ability to hold. Together, as one, they stay consciously present to see the alchemical change through to the end. This could be a change in relationship, the transmutation of an illness, the clearing of an ancestral wound, or the dispersing of a shadowy aspect. It takes guts, maturity, humility, and a bodhisattva's heart to stay in the eye of the storm—and to love.

> *The whole world could be choked with thorns:*
> *A lover's heart will stay a rose garden.*
> *The wheel of heaven could wind to a halt:*
> *The world of lovers will go on turning.*
> *Even if every being grew sad, a lover's soul*
> *Will still stay fresh, vibrant, light.*
> *Are all the candles out? Hand them to a lover,*
> *A lover shoots out a hundred thousand fires.*
>
> RUMI

If you are reading this quality of love, maybe a change is needed. Are you looking to transmute a stuck energy? Are you being steadfast? Are you being patient? Does your relationship require change? Are you initiating change? Have you the courage to enter the alchemical crucible? Is there a greater reality that you can hold on to when the heat is on? Transmutation happens within, but it will ultimately affect your life on the outside. Relationships will change, or they may end. One of the difficulties of leaving a relationship is letting go of the dreams you shared together. No matter whom you meet in the future, you will never share those particular dreams again. Herein lies a particular and lovely form of grief. Your dreams are dead, yet they are transmuted into infinite possibilities. When you truly embrace change and let go, you have made space for another future, be it with the same person or someone new.

Holy Prayer

—————————✦—————————

Beloved Mother Father God, help me initiate change. Help me to not fear this alchemy. Grant me the courage to be steadfast, the grace to be patient, and the heart to withstand the birthing pains of transmutation into new life. Bestow upon me the longevity required to see this through to the end and the kindness of heart to stay loving and open, to support myself completely on every level, and to offer the same to my beloved/friend/companion. Amen

⑤ Sacred Action

Transmutation requires two base elements that come together to produce a third. Our two base elements will be the light of awareness within the masculine and the emotionally mature love within the feminine.

Come together with your partner, either seated or lying down.

Close your eyes and go within.

He brings his full awareness to the situation/circumstance that requires transmutation. He is not trying to figure it out or solve it in any way—he is simply bringing light to the situation within the spaciousness of his clear and uncluttered mind.

She is holding the situation/circumstance that requires transmutation within her womb, allowing herself to feel and respond to any emotional currents of energy in a mature and grounded way. She breathes, moves, and utters sounds freely to assist the process.

Once established in your inner work, reach for one another's hands or any part of the body to make a connection, both physically and emotionally.

Feel the presence of one another in the alchemical crucible as you reassure one another by communicating through touch.

Stay present with your part of the process. Simply holding the light and being willing to feel makes miracles happen.

VIRGIN*

Virgin—a quality of beingness that is complete in itself, unsullied, untouched, and filled with luminescent innocence

The word *virgin* in this context has nothing to do with sex—that is the old paradigm understanding of the word. What we are referring to is a power, a light power of virginal innocence that sustains, teaches, and loves. The virgin power of the feminine gives everything that she is out of her own richness.

When we look at the Virgin Mary, the *real* Virgin Mary, we see an unimaginably heroic, passionate, forceful, powerful woman. No amount of humiliation, oppression, tragedy, or historical defeat could swerve her from the full *yes* she gave to the divine force who revealed her destiny.

And that woman, through the absolute abandon of her surrender to the unfolding of her destiny, became one with the motherhood of God, uniting the depths of her humanity with the depths of divinity found within the Great Mother. That is the real Mary, and that, Beloved

---

*This pearl, which is mainly directed toward women, is parallel to the Pillar pearl (page 153), which is mainly directed toward men. Of course everyone can gain from reading and absorbing the importance of both pearls for the masculine and feminine essences inside all of us.

Friend, is the quality of virgin light power that we too must open to for this same transfiguration to occur.

The virgin power has returned once again in our midst, and, as before, she returns at a pivotal time in our evolution. This virgin power within us finds the courage to yet again set sail on a course of transfiguration that can truly be described as heroic. The virgin within us is ennobled by a sacred divine pride—she knows that through her own essential vessel a great love force is destined to stream through her children and transform the planet.

This is an amazing power, and it is a model for all beings that question the magnitude of this work. There are times when we may feel defeated by the craziness and madness of this world—and this is the time to turn to the virgin. Within her radiance, within your *own* radiance, you will come to realize the true meaning of the *magnificat*—the endless grace streaming forth into the one who is brave enough, wild enough, and surrendered enough to embrace the full splendor and power of the virgin light power, to incarnate it, and to give his or her whole life to it.

Not only is she proud and delighted to be orchestrating this great force, she *is* this great force as she burns with ecstatic joy.

Holy Prayer

———————✦———————

Beloved Mother Father God, lead me to my virgin light power. Help me to discover the blessed radiance of my yes fully and completely. Grant me the courage to dissolve all distractions and dilutions from that yes so I may magnify Your presence. Help me radiate and multiply the frequency of my virgin power so that it shines so brightly within and without. Let me burn with ecstatic joy and come alive only with Your undulating truth. Do not allow me to dilute or cheapen the vibrancy within me. Lead me directly into a life that will stand beside the Virgin Mother's in honor and authenticity. Amen.

✺ Sacred Action

Beloved One, make your home in the breath as you begin to meditate on that young girl in Nazareth who receives news from an angel of what she is destined to be and what she is destined to birth. Identify yourself with that possibly frightened, but heroic little girl. Identify with the frightened and courageous little girl or boy within you—because that is the place that surrenders and flows with heroism. Within the Virgin Mother's womb, which is connected to your own, your own Christ consciousness will be born.

When you have identified yourself with her, pray to her to give you the courage to say "Yes—be it done to me according to thy word."

And really, honestly, fervently say those words again and again as a mantra, and each time you say them go deeper into what they truly mean. Connect with what they are asking you to change, with what they are asking you to face, with what they are asking you to let go of. Connect with what they're asking you to incarnate in the core of your life.

If you do this practice for twenty minutes in the morning and twenty minutes at night for 40 days, something will become very real to you, and you will begin to taste yourself as the virgin with an immaculate purity within you longing to be fully born. And the mystery of the deep, deep role of the sacred feminine in the birth of the Christ consciousness won't become intellectual to you but unbelievably, nakedly, gloriously, and amazingly real.

ALCHEMICAL BODY PRACTICE
MEETING THE TANTRIC MARY, VIRGIN MARY, AND MYSTICAL MARY

We believe Mary, in all of her aspects, is the fullness of the Great Divine Mother. It is no surprise that the Christed story contains these three aspects of the feminine—the tantric, the virgin, and the mystic. At the core of every evolutionary shift upon this planet—in every classical epoch and golden civilization—we find these three aspects, because she *is* the evolutionary shift. It is through her body that we are reborn. And if we chose to be reborn gracefully—then we must come to know her with every cell of our being, both intimately and abstractly.

Tantric Mary

Mary Magdalene is the tantric aspect of the Great Mother. She is the one who keeps the great tantric and erotic mysteries. Within her body of work we come to know how human thought and emotion has the power to expand and ascend to its origin by the practice of sexual holiness. It is not enough to know the varying facts and history of Mary Magdalene. We must know her essence. The gateway she holds open is for those who wish to know by experiencing the feeling states of erotic love. Mary Magdalene not only radiated the Divine Presence; she augmented it, and she still does. She fully experienced the Divine Presence in Sacred Relationship at the most edgy and incandescent levels. She was prepared to go to the depths of the Mystery and to the depths of desire to find the gold that can be lifted from that dark boiling cauldron and offer up that gold to the Divine.

Only through the restoration of the divine eros as the alchemical, transfiguring force of the birth, can we really come to know her. Yet we have to go one step further, for none of this can be known through the mind. Mary Magdalene's soul lived this alchemy with such abandoned, pure, naked love in the midst of devastating heartbreak. Her love with Yeshua was a mutually empowered gift in the name of the holy, in the name of the great work of the Divine. That can be the image that burns in your heart when you come to know Mary Magdalene. For she is both divine and human—a being who is astonishingly beautiful, creative, transformative, and evolutionary at the highest, most intense levels of nakedness, tenderness, wildness, and truth.

Virgin Mary

Mother Mary is the virgin aspect of the Great Mother. Through her absolute surrender to the unfolding of her destiny, she became one with the motherhood of God, uniting the depths of her humanity with the depths of the Divinity of the Mother.

Her virginity has nothing to do with having sex or not. It

represents an unsullied, vast cosmic love fire that *is* the Divine Feminine, complete in itself. This force will get through any obstacle; it will survive any attempt at pollution or manipulation. It is the fire force at the center of the Universe that is virgin, and this woman has been and still is honored by the heroic flame of that pure, indomitable, rapturous, powerful, and creative love fire. This is the full virgin force—an aspect of the Divine Feminine we are being hurtled toward.

Mystic Mary

The Black Madonna is the Mystic aspect of the Great Mother. She is the queen of the dark void, queen of the shadow, queen of the dark night, and queen of the destruction-creation process. She is the birthing force of the divinized self through the absolute dismantling of the false self and every illusion. She instigates destruction, walks alongside you in your sorrow, takes you through the valley of death, and rebirths you as a clear and true Christed being. She is powerful. She does not take "no" for an answer, especially if you have previously said, "yes, yes, yes!"

Know that she is the force of the Dark Mother and learn to bow to her. She holds open the mystical gateway to gnosis—know thyself. When we look at the Christ story, the Black Madonna is the crucifixion and resurrection aspect of this path. She is the humiliation, the exile, the abandonment—*and* the rebirth. Not for one second are you alone, for the Dark Mother is right alongside you—although it will feel as if she isn't. And that is her gift.

Let us now prepare to meet these three aspects and bring them into the oneness of their absolute truth. The following sacred practices are adapted from visions that I (Anaiya) experienced that shook me free of all of the conditionings that I had inherited about Mary—whether in her form as Mary Magdalene, Mother Mary, or the Black Madonna. I hope these practices will enable you to integrate this knowledge and to prepare you for this great evolutionary journey that I believe she is fully orchestrating.

Ŝ *Meeting the Tantric Mary*

Imagine now that you are going to meet the tantric Mary in some Bedouin tent deep in the blazing heart of the Sinai desert.

You are on a camel, following one of her gloriously handsome brothers into the desert at sunset. When you arrive at a beautifully decorated tent, aglow with flickering amber candlelight, the soft pulse of exotic music caresses your ears. The gorgeous man dismounts his camel and helps you down from yours. There is a twinkle in his eyes that delights and enchants you. He offers his arm to escort you to the billowing entrance of the tent. He leads you inside, saying, "Welcome, Beloved, take a seat and make yourself at home. She will be with you shortly."

The rich, pungent vapor of spikenard fills your nostrils. You turn to follow the scent, when suddenly you see her. She is a stunning vision in red; a gorgeous, rapturous beauty encased in brown velvety skin with tumbling chestnut curls. You stand in the presence of Mary Magdalene, a powerful blend of sensual erotica and heartfelt kindness. Her smile fills the tent and your heart.

She welcomes you, and in her vibrant embrace you get to hold and touch the pulsating throb of her life force and her great depth of being. As you close your eyes in this embrace, you seem to enter another world, where you find her yet again. She is with you on the inside and on the outside.

You find yourself sitting down and asking, "Mary, show me how I may embody your tantric holiness. How do I love with the whole of my body?"

And with that, she brings you deep into the mystery of your meditation and heartfelt prayer. She shares with you, at a pace you are ready for, everything you desire to know . . .

Ŝ *Meeting the Virgin Mary*

Imagine now that you are going to meet the Virgin Mary at her home in the foothills of Mt. Koressos, just outside Ephesus in Turkey.

As you walk along the cobbled streets toward her front door, you notice how modest her home is. Simplicity and peace radiate through the stone walls of this humble dwelling, yet it feels so rich and divine that it seems to wrap its arms around you.

As you approach the door on a walkway through the garden, a benevolent, huge tabby cat crosses your path and playfully rubs the side of his belly against your leg as he purrs and meows. The garden is filled with an abundance of flowers, fruits, and vegetables as well as comfortable chairs where you can rest and enjoy the beauty of the natural world.

Just as you are about to knock on the door, it opens. A woman's voice calls to you "Come in, Beloved! Make your way toward the kitchen." You tentatively walk through the house, noticing the numerous vases of roses on every shelf, table, and niche. There is a sense of delight and luminosity everywhere. You feel safe—so palpably safe that all the fears you have ever carried dissolve to dust.

A glow emanates from the kitchen combined with the warm smell of freshly baked cinnamon and nutmeg bread. You walk forward and see the glorious, luminous, white silhouette of the Madonna. She is pure, loving light radiating far beyond her kitchen, into the world. Her mercy and peace almost bring you to your knees, and in her presence you feel completely redeemed and forgiven for all you have done throughout all your lifetimes. She sees your face, and in her kindness, she lowers her light so that she does not blind your eyes. Then slowly she comes before you, extending her hand as she says, "Welcome daughter/son—I have been expecting you."

You find yourself taking her hand and asking, "Mary, show me what virgin power is. How may I come to embody it?"

And with that, she brings you deep into the mystery of your meditation and heartfelt prayer. She shares with you, at a pace you are ready for, everything you desire to know . . .

§ Meeting the Mystical Mary

> *This path to the primordial religious experience . . . is like*
> *a still small voice, and it sounds from afar. It is ambiguous,*
> *questionable, dark, presaging dangerous and hazardous*
> *adventure; a razor-edged path to be trodden for God's sake*
> *only, without assurance and without sanction.*
>
> CARL JUNG, *THE ARCHETYPES*
> *AND THE COLLECTIVE UNCONSCIOUS*

Imagine now that you are going to meet the Black Madonna in a sacred cave deep in the heartlands of Southern France. You find yourself being guided by a local who just *happens* to know which cave she is residing in. The track is narrow and seems hardly used, although every so often there is a pile of rocks that signals you're on the right path.

You start to feel the sheer power of the mountain, and it suddenly takes your breath away. The guide notices this and holds you gently by the elbow as you both look back on the path that you have come by. You gasp out loud—you had no idea how high you had climbed! The guide whispers to you, "This is known as the Valley of Fire, the most active mountain range in the south of France for telluric activity. That's the reason why she is here."

After another heart-pounding climb, you are at the mouth of the cave—a gaping black oval that is both warm and foreboding. "That's as far as I go," says the guide. "The rest you do by yourself. She is in there. She knows you are coming." With that, the guide turns and walks away.

Your heart is still hammering, your breath is shallow, and your legs feel frozen. After talking yourself into it, you walk inside the cave. It is pure blackness. Your eyes cannot see anything, and despite adjusting to the darkness, your night vision does not appear. This is more than darkness; it is . . . black light.

And still you keep walking slowly into the blackness, when suddenly in front of you there is breath upon your face and a hand reaching for yours. With your other hand you reach out and immediately come into contact with a body. Glued to the spot, you realize she is here. The Black Madonna stands before you.

Her voice comes from the depths of velvety darkness. "I am here. You asked to meet me. How may I serve the awakening of your soul, Beloved Child of the Christed Heart?"

Her words rebound within you, opening and awakening all the dimensional places and spaces in which you reside. You feel yourself merging with her blackness as you take her hand and speak. "Black Madonna, reveal in me the mystery that you hold. How may I come to embody it?"

And with that, she brings you deep into the mystery of your meditation and heartfelt prayer. She shares with you, at a pace you are ready for, everything you desire to know . . .

WISDOM

Wisdom—an experience of total absorption into the Absolute that is beyond the intellect and that reveals total insight

Wisdom is the name and essence of the Holy Sophia, who is not a deity, but an aspect of the Divine Presence. She is mostly associated with the Shekinah, known as the Holy Spirit in Christianity, and known in some form throughout all cultures and traditions as the indwelling presence. In the Kabbalah and other mystical works of medieval times, the Shekinah is often treated as the consort of God who can only be reunited with God through human fulfillment of the Great Work, or Restoration.

In our times mystics are stewards of this essence, this wisdom. What is a mystic? Who are these wise fools among us? Contrary to popular perception, a mystic is not a magician or a crystal ball gazer. Rather, a mystic is a person who has had an experience of God's love so unmistakable that it changes him or her forever, imparting a confidence that cannot be shaken, a humility that cannot be doubted, a freedom that exudes love, a gentleness, and an authenticity. A mystic knows from experience, not books, that we are each beautiful beyond our understanding, loved beyond our capacity to love, united beyond our perceptions of difference and separation. For me, a mystic is one who longs for an all-embodied and ever encompassing stream of wisdom that delights, deepens, and extends out into the world as pure, unsullied radiance.

A mystical experience is one of the gifts of the Holy Sophia, imparting wisdom—an experience of total absorption into the Absolute that is beyond the intellect and that reveals total insight. It is an experience that the mystic, in contemplation, continuously longs for within. All spiritual and religious teachings have an esoteric, mystical path—including this teaching of Sacred Relationship.

The mystic within us longs to become swallowed up in a unifying consciousness that is greater than our own. This is the experience of wisdom. The mystic loves God, both the transcendent and immanent expressions, as a devotional lover whose love is not only intimate, but also personal. In our sacred relationships it is simply not enough to *read* about how to make our relationship holy—we must seek out the actual experience of it with a hunger and relentless longing that transcends our human love into divine, unconditional love.

Holy Prayer

---✦---

Beloved Mother Father God, You are my beloved, and I long to know how far and wide my love can grow. Without You I live in the darkness with no ray of light. Your love gives power to my life, beautifying my soul so it can be consumed in Your delicious flame of kindness and vast expansion. I want all of You, more than anything. Teach me, Beloved, teach me to love without fear, limitation, restriction, or distrust. I need to be reckless in my love for You; I long to gaze upon You with a thousand eyes and drink in Your aching beauty. Help me turn to every aspect of Your creation and express my love in every conceivable delightful, joyful, wild way! Amen.

§ *Sacred Action*

Are you missing the love of God? Are you approaching this work as a theory, as something to learn, rather than something to live? Have you become too serious, too intellectual? If so, I invite you to open to wisdom.

Beloved, let us take this time together to enter the cloud of unknowing, a practice of silent prayer and meditation. Allow yourself the time to drop into a true and honest ignorance of God, not as a form of unworthiness, but from a simple and honest truth—that we do not truly know what or who God is, what God looks like, or even what God actually does.

Allow yourself to *not know* any spiritual ideas, concepts, or teachings, apart from one—God is love. Simply drop into meditation and allow the feeling sensations of your soul to move toward God. Have a feeling communion—your essence touching God's essence.

Drop into your breath—and ask yourself, are you breathing or are you being breathed?

Contemplate one of the greatest mystical truths, that your breath *is* the Holy Spirit. This is God's way of not only penetrating you, but comforting you.

And then, allow yourself to be transported into a mystical world of experience that cannot be spoken of, only experienced, as you ask one last simple question: "Beloved Holy Sophia, show me the true nature of [my choices, feelings, circumstances, thoughts, crisis, health condition, etc.]." And allow the wisdom to flow.

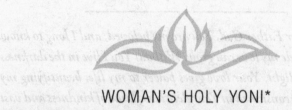

WOMAN'S HOLY YONI*

Yoni—the vulva, a symbol of divine procreative energy

The labia, the lips of love, form the entrance to the yoni. They are guardians not just of the body and sexuality, but also of your soul. They are the flowering sentinels who serve your sacred well and life force, and whose message is *I honour myself.* They hold the following soul qualities: welcoming, safety, trust, honor, praise, appreciation, connection to the web of life, warmth, wholesomeness, divine desire, and giving and receiving of love.

The sacred gate of the yoni flowers with praise and appreciation. Once a woman honors and appreciates herself, she can receive divine procreative energy from another through her yoni. When you are truly recognized and seen, you will feel welcomed by life. Then your yoni will become a welcoming portal to any energy you deem worthy of entrance. Respecting this sacred gate with true self love heals you of many life experiences relating to sexuality, your father, or past lovers.

---

*This pearl, which is mainly directed toward women, is parallel to the Man's Holy Lingam pearl (page 148), which is mainly directed toward men. Of course everyone can gain from reading and absorbing the importance of both pearls for the masculine and feminine essences inside all of us.

Vulnerability and humility open the doorway to love and intimacy. Without vulnerability and humility, as well as appreciation and devotion, the yoni can never open, and the grail womb cannot be entered. Remember, intimacy is a mutual exchange—in giving these qualities, we receive them.

The entrance to the yoni helps open us into deeper trust. Trust yourself and what you are letting into you *or* choosing to keep out. The wounds women carry here, both personal and collective, revolve around trust. For men to come fully into the yoni they must approach women with appreciation and purity of heart and intent, completely honoring this sacred portal into the feminine. They must also feel welcomed in order to enter the yoni this way.

For a woman to surrender into this space of trust she must respect her partner and feel held, safe, and supported with him. She must trust both his strength and gentleness as well as his ability to penetrate her with love. Of course she will not surrender or open the sacred yoni gate if she does not feel respect and appreciation from the man she is with.

Sadly, the nature of relationship today has led to a forgetting of this. Confused in the collective unconscious fog left by the abuse perpetrated for centuries, women and young girls have forgotten how sacred this portal really is. Most women hold a great unconscious sadness at the loss of their connection to the power of true feminine surrender, which is accessed through the lips of love in a relationship of trust. Sacred safety occurs in the body when we magnetically and emotionally—not just intellectually or wishfully—believe that we are truly safe, welcomed, honored, and appreciated by our partners. Our womb and bodies know this, yet our minds will often deceive us.

If a man sexually enters a woman without respect, without loving connection—shoving the penis in for his own pleasure and self-gratification—sex can be identified with violence, ownership, conquering, animal aggression, or plain lust. Every time this has happened to you, it is recorded on the delicate fabric of your yoni lips and as a remembrance within your soul.

By allowing these actions, women lose their sense of beauty and sanctity, their sense of being cherished. Gradually their feminine awareness, intuition, sensitivity, and magnetic-feeling self diminishes. Their feminine power, based on the body, sexuality, emotions, and God, begins to slip and fade away. Their sense of inner safety, trust, and vulnerability recedes as numbness sets in. The lips become desensitized to true intimacy, and many women have little feeling beyond this gate.

In the new paradigm that conscious men and women are co-creating, the yoni gate must become fully honored and vibrantly alive. A woman in her true power is the Goddess incarnate—fully healed of sexual wounds and repression. Her beloved is likewise fully empowered and healed. Actually, the word *yoni* means more than simply the body parts called labia and vulva; *yoni* in the original Sanskrit has many meanings and represents the divine passage for body and soul, the holder, the matrix of generation, the origin or primal source of all creation, the birthplace of the Universe! In Vedic astrology each child is considered to be born from a *yoni of stars*—the constellations that prevailed during the child's birth.

The yoni is a temple gate, where the pure essence of a woman can be connected with. It is the opening into the holy womb, the birth space for all life. The yoni is a great teacher, for a woman learns true self-love, sovereignty, and self-respect by welcoming into her oni *only* that which is loving, trustworthy, and honoring of her essence. The yoni is the sacred doorway into a woman's holiest of places.

After reciting the prayer below, visualize, breathe, and feel all the emotions releasing from your yoni lips, like rings of black smoke. Visualize your yoni lips filled with a beautiful pink-magenta color. Feel these colors and breathe them in as they regenerate and massage your yoni lips.

Holy Prayer

✦

Beloved Mother Father God, Please help me feel and release all my feelings of anger, resentment, and bitterness against all males; all my feelings of shame, guilt, or rejection; and my deepest feelings of unworthiness, humiliation, or sadness. Please help me completely release all of this from my yoni and soul! I desire to be a Queen of the new paradigm, birthing the new age of divinity within myself and in all men as well. Empower my creative and sexual beingness with Your expansion! Infuse my yoni with Your divine procreative energy, so I may bring my heart's presence into the act of love. Amen.

⑤ Sacred Action

Pay attention to your yoni. Is this a part of you that you have abandoned? For a lingam, entering a healed yoni it is like entering silk: smooth, soft, juicy, inviting, and disposed to love's sensitivity and slowness, as opposed to lust, agitation, or violence. Making love is unhurried, luxuriating in its sensitivity to movements of love, light ,and sublimated passion. The velvet softness of your internal, intimate temple softly closes around the supple divine lingam, drawing it in ever deeper through your opening blooming heart, through your breath, through your magnetism, through the subtlest of movements, through your desire for God through your open heart and womb. Is this how you feel about your yoni?

Place your fingers slowly, gently, and lovingly, with conscious attention, at the lips of your yoni. Simply feel her: the texture, the warmth, the contours, and the feeling of the skin.

Gently cup both your hands over your yoni, connecting with your heart and praying for the Great Mother to imbue your yoni and womb with her presence as you whisper these words:

> *Beloved Yoni, I truly appreciate you.*
> *I love you.*
> *I respect you, even if I did not in the past.*
> *You are beautiful, loving, and kind. You can heal, nurture, and*
> *   transform.*
> *You are a valuable part of me.*
> *I honor you from the depths of my heart.*
> *Beloved One, please lead me to my sensual sacred self.*
> *Open so deeply so I may surrender and let go.*
> *From this moment on, I allow only love to enter me.*

If you feel any emotions arise, simply breathe into them and allow yourself to feel.

Keep repeating the above words until you believe them.

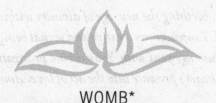

WOMB*

Womb—the container of divine procreative energy that births both physical and non-physical offspring

Part of our original innocence is found in our sexuality, and we all have to do our sexual healing. At the beginning we may read some books, engage in prayer and meditation, or try out some neo-tantric exercises. However, as the journey continues we will have to commit to a deeper practice, one that involves the body and the flow of pure awakened love. For deeper sexual wholeness to come alive, one has to love with soul and with God. This is why most forms of tantra can never fully authenticate the journey: our heart needs to be profoundly and powerfully connected to our sexuality. The new paradigm also recognizes that God must be included in the bedroom too! Old paradigm ideas that sexuality is dirty or sinful must be jettisoned out the window. This is ever more apparent at this time in Earth's evolution, when so many twin flames, or beloved couples, are reuniting.

For the journey of sexual healing to be complete, certain elements are essential. There needs to be trust—deep trust. There needs to be love, both erotic and divine love. And there needs to be God, not some off-planet deity or abstract field, but a real, live soul of Father-Mother who is a beloved, for the waves of longing, ecstasy, and devotion to awaken into a boiling cauldron of rapturous illumination and obliteration. Once this journey begins to take shape and form, then one finds oneself entering the womb—the deep, primordial blackness that contains the mystical elements of sexuality and its unspoken doorway into other dimensions and realms of existence.

---

*This pearl, which is mainly directed toward women, is parallel to the Generator pearl (page 129), which is mainly directed toward men. Of course everyone can gain from reading and absorbing the importance of both pearls for the masculine and feminine essences inside all of us.

The womb beckons the man upon a journey—a journey that promises new life and wholeness, in exchange for his worldly status and material forgetfulness. As the womb awakens and becomes part of the woman's sexual nature, its natural magnetic pulse of life will draw the essence of the man into its center. And he will want to go there; all men desire to go there. Whether men *allow* themselves to go there is a different matter, as the all-enfolding, all-engulfing presence of the womb swallows all into its black velvety vastness. Yet a centered and conscious man has much to gain from a journey into the sacred womb.

When the man and woman surrender within themselves and allow this innate drawing inward, back into the source of life and original innocence, to occur, they will enter an infinite space together. Together both partners, while in the opened womb space, will pass within its infinite reaches. Much of what they have known will be annihilated in this sweet innocence merged with passion; nothing of the past can be present here. The old tried and tested ways of making love are abandoned, as something new and fresh is touched for the first time. This sacred touch creates life and vitality in a previously dormant cave. One realizes that before this moment, one has never truly felt the vastness of pure and sincere love combined with sexuality, despite the sexual adventures one may have experienced. The touch may be tender at first, as the womb's virginity is paradigm altering; but what is now being revealed and opened changes lovemaking forever.

As a woman, your womb is your grounding center for love, your firm foundation for true feminine soul gravity, a woman's sacred center in union with her heart. It is your inner well of creativity and creation. Your womb is part of your feminine soul essence embodied here on Earth, deep within the human form. It is a woman's most reliable, trusted, and safe *home*.

The womb holds the seed of your being, your first creative spark, and the infinite potential of the living void. Ultimately the womb leads you to the womb of all life—the Galactic Center—and beyond, to the space through which all of life travels in the process of manifesting from the formless.

When you realize this experientially, you can begin to create within your own womb, placing your heart's desires within its field to be birthed into the world and into yourself.

The womb will only open herself to a man if she fully trusts, respects, and admires him and feels like she can surrender into his masculine presence and role as generator. The womb will only open if she feels she can be guided by him safely and fully let go with him. This is not a mental decision—this comes from the primordial, instinctual knowing of the womb and one's deep heart knowing.

As you say the following holy prayer with full feeling, rub your hands together until they are warm. Place your fingers together in an inverted pyramid shape, slowly, with conscious attention, on your womb. Simply feel here, and drop your feeling heart consciousness deep down into her. Gently breathe down deep into her through pursed lips, deeper and deeper. Allow yourself to drop down into womb consciousness.

Holy Prayer

✦

Beloved Mother Father God, I am now ready to fully embody my womb and awaken its mystical wisdom. Orchestrate around me the initiations into the hidden depths of the Sacred Feminine so I may release all the wounds that have shut down and dampened my womb's radiance. Empower my womb with Your warm expansion from the ever-present realm! Infuse my womb with Your divine procreative energy, so I may be able to bring all of my being into the act of love. I want to embody the tantric, virgin, and mystic within me. I am ready to be a Queen of the new paradigm, birthing the new age of divinity within myself and all life. Help me to feel and release all past hurts— with men as well as anger, mistrust, fear of survival, fear of dying, fear of truly living, my feelings of being unsupported, my deep feelings of loneliness, my lack of appreciating and nurturing myself, my self-judgment and self-punishment, all blame, my need for approval, and my deep feelings of grief and sadness. Help me release them all from my womb and soul. Amen.

⑤ Sacred Action

Beloved One, pour some almond oil into your hands as you rub them together. Visualize a blazing orange ball of light between your hands as you place them over your womb in an inverted pyramid shape, sinking the orange light deep into the depths of your womb. Breathe into your womb powerfully through your mouth, and with each breath feel this orange light intensify in brightness and power, spinning and radiating through your womb, body, emotions, and energy field, dissolving negative feelings, memories, and images.

After breathing this way for a while, say: "Beloved Mother God, Divine Healing Intelligence, please send 4,000 percent orange ray of purification into my womb!"

Sound and tone the three syllables of Om—Ahhh-Oooo-Mmmm—deep into your womb, repeating this for a few minutes. Circulate and connect the sound and breath together so it is one continuous flow. Allow the sound to gently penetrate deep within. Travel with the sound deeper and deeper. (You can do the toning silently if you prefer.)

When you are deep in the womb, pray:

I so appreciate You, Beloved Mother God, for my life. Thank You, Mother, for my body. Thank You, Mother, for my world and thank You, Mother, for everyone and everything in it. Thank You for Your divine love. Beloved Mother God, please install, activate, and anchor the perfect human blueprint for the womb of love into me now. I love You.

BOOK OF TRUTH

Attributes of the Divine Masculine

I Am: Pure Consciousness.

I Am the Generator, Orchestrator, and Power of Truth. Source of Guidance, Full of Drive and Intelligence. Fearless, Discerning, Decisive, and Giving, I Honor the Beloved with my Devoted Pillar of Commitment.

I Am Sovereign, King who serves all, Father, Lover, Divine Man.

I Am a Lingam of Light.

I Am Fulfilled and Free, a Rhythmic, Primordial Power of Light

I Am the Actions of Man as the Son of My Father, Intelligence of Transcendent Love, and Formless Truth: I Am Enlightenment.

The truth of Divine Masculine power has nothing to do with what the world calls "power." It has nothing to do with rule or control. This power amounts to a total revolution of every patriarchal notion of power, status, and worth. True Divine Masculine power is free from hierarchy; it is unrelated to the old guru system and it repudiates any claim to the myth that high spiritual attainment entitles one to wield power over others. True masculine power is steady yet flowing, disciplined yet wild, joyfully free and uncensored, peaceful yet powerful, and a humble and grand commitment to be who one is in a male form and from this place serve all beings with the love of a great Father. This true Divine Masculine energy is arising in tandem with the return of Divine Feminine, and birthing a new paradigm of united love, wisdom, and power on the planet.

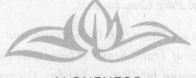

ALONENESS

Aloneness—all one in solitude and inner silence

Aloneness is a time to reflect, integrate, and contemplate. All of us need our cave, our inner sanctum where we can replenish, rejuvenate, and gain a fresh energy and perspective on what life has been delivering to us. The masculine part of us thrives on solitude, where all parts can regather, commune, and emerge anew.

Being alone is being all-one. You silently sound a call for yourself to hear the voice of the soul and relax all parts of yourself into wholeness. This is a redemptive act: to recollect and reunite all parts of yourself around the pillar of the One.

In this gathering, we recollect ourselves and return to our source, our original wholeness. Aloneness gives you an opportunity to hear your true nature, the still, small voice within, that always *knows*. This voice, always present, follows the guidance of your pure soul in all situations.

This still, small voice within serves to bring you into divine will, which serves love. Surrendering to divine will allows our highest potential to manifest. It wants only the best for us. Often we do not know what is best for us, what will lead us to true joy and happiness and the strength of unspeakable peace.

When we flow with divine will, it releases us from the compulsive need to do, and we surrender to what is happening in our present experience of life right now. We see that our identity, our sense of value, our love, our strength, and our peace do not depend on doing.

Divine will is most deeply felt and understood when you are alone. You can hear it better!

Aloneness is a soothing balm that welcomes deeper, softer emotions within you, gently, gradually, easing and cradling your heart in this tender flow. As Hafiz shares in his poem "Absolutely Clear," "Don't surrender your loneliness so quickly. Let it cut more deep. Let it ferment and season you as few human or even divine ingredients can."

Loneliness, sadness, tenderness and deep healing happen in the heart sitting in solitude. Our deepest pain, our need for love that has not been met and fulfilled, arises. We feel it, we surrender to its sacred tears, and we become a little bit more whole.

> *Only those people who are capable of being alone are capable of love, of sharing, of going into the deepest core in the other person—without possessing the other, without becoming dependent on the other, without reducing the other to a thing, and without becoming addicted with the other. They allow the other absolute freedom, because they know that if the other leaves, they will be as happy as they are now. Their happiness cannot be taken by the other, because it is not given by the other.*
>
> OSHO, *NEW MAN FOR THE NEW MILLENNIUM*

Many of us are scared of true connection and true relationship because we have not truly connected with certain parts of ourselves. In connecting with our newly discovered aspects we can also let go of security devices and strategies that we have built as crutches for walking in the world, which all prevent us from being open, transparent, and living in trust with self, other, and life itself. In feeling seen, our isolated aloneness can dissipate into forgiveness and closeness.

When you are willing to experience the depths of aloneness, you will discover connection everywhere. Turning to face your fear, you meet the warrior who lives within. Opening to your loss, you gain embrace. Each condition you flee from will pursue you. Each condition you welcome will transform you.

Aloneness and true silence is a powerful force that can carve us open. As Mooji has often shared in his satsangs, "Only when you can face and bear your own silence will you be free." Silence and stillness happen in mind, body, and soul. In the mind, everything ceases. The body finally rests. The soul takes its rightful place as ruler, and you are allowed to be the hero.

Silence cannot be forced. From the souls feeling wisdom, silence occurs when your emotions are felt, released, and brought into wholeness. Any emotional disturbance still left in you manifests as the inability to go into silence. This is quite different from the mind's (or spirit's) perspective, which can train and use its willpower to go into quietness and realms of light, bliss, and power. As the soul is master of the spirit, and spirit is the vehicle of soul, true silence rests in simply having no emotional healing left to do within you.

Solitude, when you are alone and without any human contact at all for a period of time, can center you in your deeper self. Science has shown that your brainwaves change after seventy-two hours in Nature, without other humans or electrical interference, such as Internet, phones, or electricity. Your mood changes, becomes lighter, more connected, more rounded. Your mind-set relaxes and you feel yourself again, without interference, emotional resonance, or vibrational information from others. You can rest in yourself at last.

Your DNA is constantly emitting, emanating, and vibrating information from its spiral helixes into your body, mind, soul, environment, and other people in your immediate surroundings. While you are reading these words, your DNA is doing this. Going into solitude in Nature, alone, brings forth a wonderful invitation to resonate only with yourself and find out more of who you are and what stuff you are made of.

Holy Prayer

✦

Beloved Father Mother God, help me feel my fears about being alone, and help me do it anyway. Help me rest more into myself. Help me gently become more of who I am. Help me to value aloneness and solitude and to seek out regular time in Your Holy Presence. I love You! Amen.

၆ Sacred Action

Beloved One, take time today to be alone, even if it is for ten minutes in the garden.

Put your phone and computer away, and just sit down and do nothing.

Take time every day to be alone in Nature without anything or anyone.

Enjoy this alone time. Rest in your breathing.

Wouldn't you like more?

CONSCIOUSNESS

Consciousness—the state of being aware of and witnessing all of oneself in all things

All your atoms are essentially empty space. *You* are a black hole, and black holes lie in each and every one of your cells. *You* are rotating fields of energy housing emptiness. Nothing here, nothing there. This empty space is potentially infinite, and it is what *you* are.

Infinite spaciousness. Eternal rest. No identity to support, no security to fall back on. Neither this, nor that. Not this way, not that way. What is eternal? It is not this, or that, as both are temporary, transient, fleeting moments in time and space. What is there to hold on to? What can give you support? What is this *you* that needs all these things?

In the void of pure consciousness, gone is the world, gone is yourself, gone is the dream and serving it, gone is all you have ever realized, achieved, and hoped for. Gone is shadow, gone is family, gone is clinging. Gone is lower self, gone is higher self, gone are guides. Gone is mind, gone is body, gone is my location, gone is my orientation, gone is my position in life. Gone are all things that define you. Gone is right and wrong, gone are all needs and meanings, gone are all layers and vanity, gone is death and fear. In the void of pure consciousness one's idea of soul and different layers of body dissolve and are surrendered. One's essence, so valued and treasured, used as the reference point for your movements and aspirations in life, is left behind, burnt in the fire of nothing.

One's position and ways of mapping out one's position in life go. Gone is the fear of death in all its forms, and gone is the need to ascribe meaning to any and all occurrences in creation. There is no emotion. It is what it is. Your life, past and present, has nothing to it. There is no sense of achievement. Instead there is just light, clarity, and love. There is no judgment of anything. One moves beyond the rules and laws of creation and therefore masters them completely.

Expressing nothing from nothing means there is nothing to hold on to, no belief, path, or teaching to give or for others to follow and create another series of beliefs, dogmas, or heroes out of. You are the hero, and this is your journey, a journey that ends when all is gone, on all levels, in all situations.

As the layers of self dissolve, as the veils of thought and emotion dissolve in the fire of nothing, one is left with nowhere to go, nothing to be, nothing to grasp at, nothing to fill. With no *I,* all conflict ceases, and we act in the underlying current of reality, which knows what to do and when to do it. All is surrendered and the soul self finishes its journey, a journey that begins and ends. Pure consciousness never began and never will end.

If you need someone or something to validate who you are, then you and the other are both creating a consensual image that has no reality. Returning to the source and origin of everything allows us to know who we really are and what everything is. Naked truth arises.

You are part of it all; it is part of you. It is not a static space, but a potent, whole emptiness teeming with infinite possibilities. It is not pure as it is not impure, as there is nothing within it to change, wither, die, or mutate. It cannot increase or decrease: it is always ever same. All a human can do is continually relax all that is not this within him or her.

There is no judgment, right or wrong, in emptiness, nothing to measure a self against another self. There is no comparison, no contrast, nothing to get. It goes nowhere and comes from nowhere. What always is here is always here: it is just all the thoughts, needs, and sense of self that obscure the underlying reality of what never changes and what has never been created.

What has been created always changes and dies. What has never been created cannot go anywhere or cease to be.

Holy Prayer

———————✦———————

Beloved Father Mother God, help me relax into the void of pure consciousness. Help me release and embrace all parts of myself so I can enter Your womb of total rebirth. Help me enter the space between all spaces. Help me let go of myself. Beloved Mother Father God, grant me the presence to witness my thoughts and emotions this day. Help me feel what I have to feel and witness what no longer serves me. Help me no longer be a victim of the swirling currents of my own need for love. Help me stand in who I am. Amen.

ᕯ Sacred Action

Beloved One, are you feeling exhausted by your mind and emotions? Do you feel as if you have been thrust into an ocean of commotion as you are tossed and turned by a hungry tide of thoughts and feelings?

Take a deep breath, Dearest Friend, and imagine there is no such thing as words and language. Imagine there are no sensations or dialogue that could possibly describe your thoughts. Imagine . . . you are totally innocent.

Now look at an object, right in front of you. Just gaze at it, without any labeling of what it is, what you have thought it to be, or even what it could be. Look at it as if you have never seen it before, as if there are no words to describe it, as if it is completely new. Gaze at it in wonder.

Stay like this for a few minutes. What happens?

Now apply this process to your dilemma, to your relationship, to your challenge, and to your emotions. Innocently look upon it all, wondering, loosely with childlike curiosity.

See what happens next . . . .

DECISIVE

Decisive—making decisions clearly and effectively with our free will centered in the true self for the benefit of all

If I'm not saying "HELL YEAH!" about something, then [I] say no.

DEREK SIVERS, "NO MORE YES.
IT'S EITHER HELL YEAH! OR NO."

What stops us from decisively using our sovereign free will as innocent, joyful, and pure beings without wounds, conditioning, and need? What stops us from giving and receiving love freely without demand, expectation, and agenda? What stops us from fully loving our own self, giving our self what we fully desire, and opening to receive this from others and God?

Without need, we are free to give and receive love unconditionally. Without expectation, nothing is personal so we can be always be surprised and spontaneously touched in deep spaces with gratitude. Without agenda, it does not matter what is said or done. Without wounds, nothing hurts anymore and there are no beliefs to stop one from loving self and others.

Few souls actually use sovereign free will in a clear and decisive manner. It is a rare thing on Earth. We believe we make choices from an empowered and soulful perspective, and sometimes we do. Yet much of the time our choices are dictated by our subconscious and our conditioning. So what stops us from using sovereign free will, and why is it so rare?

Different types of spirits (entities, emotions, thoughtforms, etc.) will influence our supposed choices of our free will. Love-inspired spirits will gently try to influence you to choose more loving movements in your life. There are two forms of this influence depending on what path you are on: natural love spirits—who will guide you to change your thoughts and actions to become more successful, spiritual, and happy—and divine love spirits—who will guide you to change the very cause of your unhappiness, the condition of your soul and your emotions.

Negative (sabotaging) spirits will influence your free will by suggesting ideas, actions, and fear-based emotions that feed their sense of revenge, injustice, and pain. They may have the same wound and emotional resonance as you and will encourage you to go deeper into your vices and weaknesses, deriving a certain depraved pleasure from seeing you lose yourself in darkness. Your free will is subverted, as the negative spirits will make you believe it is your own inner voice that makes you do certain things.

Of course you are not a victim, and these spirit promptings can only arise because of a resonance and similar wound within yourself. Yet spirits regularly amplify even small things into much larger events and emotional dramas, and because you are unaware of this, your true free will is cloaked. You become possessed by a spirit and its desires. From here many things can arise: a martyr complex, fatigue, loss of personal joy, intellectualization of truth, loss of fulfillment, loss of free will, and loss of ability to progress on your soul path.

Without education about the many possibilities of choice and free will, we cannot make true decisions. Without being free of the influences that wounds generate within us, we cannot fully use free will, as our perceptions are limited to the range of awareness we live in. Outside of our own range of perceptions and awareness, nothing else exists. We live in our own filtered bubble, and our wounds are our greatest blocks to seeing reality and true being. Yet they are also our way out into freedom, true love, and sovereign free will—once healed and completed.

In the process of releasing and letting go of all these influences, we can decisively take empowered, sovereign choices into pure action. This is the last step in the chain of actualizing free will, making true decisions, and becoming a sovereign being. These actions can be radical and they can majorly impact your physical life, relationships, work, and ways of being. Making and concretely enacting these new choices will change you, fast.

Free will is one of the most powerful forces in the Universe. Through it, we choose our destiny. Choices are always available to us in each moment. Will you choose love, or something else? Gaia is a free-will planet, part of a great experiment to see what happens when we can all do whatever we want to. What do you choose?

When you are centered in deep humility, in holy desire, in all the qualities of the Divine Human, you make your choices from this place. You are centered in that self-inquiry from which true choices are made. True choice is centered in self. And it is only from this point that truly loving decisions can be made. If you are not centered here, you could make some loving choices, but you will often make unloving choices as well. Being centered in self is the absolute foundation you need to rise and bloom higher—to see with the mind of God, feel through the heart of God, and understand the mysteries of the Universe.

Holy Prayer

✦

Beloved Father Mother God, please help me make loving choices in my life. Please help me see the consequences of the decisions I make before I make them. Help me choose love over profit, convenience, and at times my own unworthiness. Help me animate the quality of decisiveness in ways that further love. Thank You. Amen.

❧ Sacred Action

Beloved One, are you feeling overwhelmed with seemingly external influences and sabotaging thoughtforms? Take this time now to make your home in your breath as you recite the prayer above and come into union with your true, most holy self. Many of our decisions are dictated by the unconscious mind. People do things without thinking about them. A shaman always contemplates his actions before doing them, seeing their chain of consequences and effects on him, others, and the world. Self-inquiry is the basis of all informed, conscious decisions.

When a decision needs to be made, do it, even if the decision is a difficult one. Stand by your decision with a powerfully unshakable presence, and others will respect this. Choose wisely, Beloved Friend, for the time of decisive action is *here*.

Essentially there are only two decisions we can make: loving ones and unloving ones. It is up to you to choose today—and every day.

DISCERNMENT

Discernment—the ability to distinguish with all senses the truth of a matter

Discernment is the beating heart of duality and reveals the unexplored parts of ourselves we sweep under the carpet. Our discernment is a hidden blessing for us to see, as it shows us what parts of ourselves still need self nurturing, compassion, and forgiveness. Discernment brings to light our greatest pains and deepest sadness.

In judgment you compare yourself to others: who is better or worse. When the wounded self is not in control, it feels threatened and fearful. We step out of truth the moment we judge, attack, defend. Forgiveness is the second most powerful force in existence, behind love. The truth is, you yourself benefit most from forgiving another or yourself as it is a sacred path to a deeper love, peace, and freedom. Being who you are in the present moment is love, and all actions done from this space are the actions of forgiveness too.

This is all possible through discernment, where we fully own the emotional sting in how we feel and view others, working toward seeing all events and people as neutral. We are open-minded about what is happening and curious about people. We choose to not judge another, realizing we make people and situations good or bad through the filters of our own wounded self.

This allows our discerning intelligence to sift through what is useful and what is not. It decides what is necessary to do in order to reach an objective. What is necessary for me to do today in order to achieve my objective of being one with God or putting my passion and desires into action in my life today?

This sifting process helps you create a new order. To enable yourself to rise to a higher order in your life, you have to dissolve the old order. You will reach a new plane of order and harmony in yourself for a while, and then you will feel a need to dissolve the old order and move to the next, higher plane of order and harmony. This process will continue throughout your life as you are evolving.

Discernment is the ability to question and look at things clearly, without emotional charge, bias, or fear. It allows one to contemplate things to see if they make logical and emotional sense, as true discernment combines both. It allows you to let go of things that can never work and persist with those things that can work because they have love as their foundation.

To be discerning we have to be self-responsible and take the reins of our reactivity. We have to be open to the other and what we are feeling and viewing. We have to be prepared to view things from a different perspective in order to gain true value from the experience. Discernment is sorting the wheat from the chaff. You sift truth from untruth. We sort out what is good for us, remembering that what is good for us today may be bad for us tomorrow.

What holds worth and value to you? What can help you on your journey? What can you do to help others in a way that is reflective of your deepest joy and gifts? What is ready to ripen within you and what is not? What do you have to nurture, and what do you leave out? What is your partner ready for, and what are you ready for?

Does your partner have the substance for you to commit to him or her? What are you both ready to commit to? What are you ready to give? What are you not ready to give or unable to give? Are you ready to give fully or do you still need healing and time in order to give? Is it the right time to take someone or something on in your life? What do you include in your expression of love, and what do you not include? What kind of relationship can you have with your partner, and is there another more worthy one for you? What obstacles stand in the way of your relationships? Are they worth navigating or not? How much time will this take? What will you have to leave out of your life, and what do you include?

Discernment is about value. What is worth your precious time, energy, and soul to invest in? Some of our giving may fall on fertile ground and be received. This brings joy. Some of our seeds of giving will fall on deaf ears and not be received, and will maybe even be judged. With discernment, one can tell who is ready for what seed, including one's self.

Discernment is about knowing yourself and your capacities right now. What you want and what you practically need to do to achieve your goals is discernment. Saving time, unnecessary heartache, and life force energy are valuable aspects of discernment, as these then free you into an accelerated path of growth, making sure you do not keep on repeating the same mistakes.

Discernment allows us to nurture and harvest our energies wisely and abundantly. It gives us space and frees up more energy to be used in fruitful ways, rather than chasing dead ends. Discernment brings efficiency, detachment, and the ability to notice an overview of our life and unfolding relatings, soul purpose jobs, and choices. No problem can ever be solved at the same level of the problem. One has to go to the next octave, beyond the problem being looked at, in order to see clearly what is possible and worthwhile, and what is not.

Holy Prayer

———————✦———————

Beloved Father Mother God, help me see the bigger picture of my life.
Help me to not judge others; help me to forgive others as You have

forgiven me. Help me look into my future with others and see whether we are both ripe for what we both want, or whether we need to go our separate ways. Thank You. Amen.

⑤ Sacred Action

Beloved One, what and who is real in your life, and what is not? What holds value and substance in your relationships? What is worth investing in, and what needs discarding? What holds value and substance within you? What is worth investing in, and what needs discarding?

Imagine you are an eagle with clear sight, soaring above your life, discerning the web of connections and commitments you live amidst. Let the eyes of discernment give you a fresh perspective.

Then write the answers to the questions posed here—straight from your clear, discerning vision. Remember, your compass of joy is a tool of discernment too.

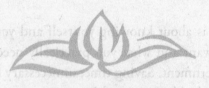

ALCHEMICAL BODY PRACTICE

DIVINE KISS

The Teacher loved her [Miriam] more than all the disciples; he often kissed her on the mouth.

THE GOSPEL OF PHILIP

The Hebrew word for kiss, *nashakh*, means "to breathe together, to share the same breath." Moreover, the word for breath is the same as the word for spirit in both Hebrew and Aramaic (*ruakh*) as well as in Greek (*pneuma*) and Latin (*spiritus*). Therefore we can say that Yeshua and Mary Magdalene shared the same breath and were united by the same spirit.

Nashakh is an ancient word found in the Old Testament. The *feeling* behind the meaning of nashakh is made clear in the "Song of Songs," a semierotic poem written by King Solomon to his beloved, the Queen of Sheba. In this context we get a tantalizing glimpse of the potential of the divine kiss, which brings our soul into the mouth and breathes our essence upon the lips of our beloved. In the nashakh we can give birth to one another by the sharing of a love so great that it marries the soul with the flesh.

While researching this subject, I (Padma) soon realized that only fragments of information still remain. Almost everything referring to the divine kiss has been burned, buried, or hidden. I found most of the information on these mystical teachings in the gnostic gospels, which, as mentioned earlier, were discovered at Nag Hammadi in 1945, though some texts have not been commonly available until the last twenty years or so. As with all the gnostic texts, the teachings are concealed from plain sight. This is not something that you learn, but something that you live. You cannot read gnostic texts and *get it* immediately with your rational mind. You have to contemplate, reflect, wonder, and pray for the deeper meaning to come to you. And come to you she does, in the form of Sophia herself—pure unadulterated wisdom.

As I turned inward to further understand these mysteries, this is what I discovered. First I must share with you the relationship I have with Yeshua and Mary, as the Word and Wisdom of the Christ Path. I understand Yeshua as being the embodiment of Logos, the Word, and Mary as the embodiment of Sophia, the Wisdom. When Yeshua would speak in Mary's presence, the word would penetrate wisdom and worlds upon worlds of experience were born.

Let that idea perfume the air between us as we continue on.

In my mind's eye, when imagining Yeshua kissing Mary on the mouth, I *saw* that he was passing her the deeper mystery behind his words through a transmission of light, breath, and love. And so, when Mary received the kiss, I *saw* her take it so deeply into her being that she came to a place brimming with fertility and creation. When this place within her received the light, love, and breath from Yeshua, she responded in wisdom and gave birth to the transmission in ways that we could all receive and understand. She translated the light into feeling, and her feeling set alight everyone surrounding her. She continues to do the same to this day.

Now let's learn how to perform the divine kiss and experience the breath that unites. The nashakh is described as a kiss between a man and woman, but it can easily be the kiss between a same-sex couple's masculine and feminine essences, and the exercises below can be used by any couple.

❧ Step One

Play some emotive background music.

Come into a cross-legged position on the floor as you sit opposite one another. Make sure the space is comfortable and that you feel supported in your seated position.

Recite "A Prayer before Union," which is found in this book on page 197.

Take this time to gently gaze upon one another, loosely holding hands, and connecting with the love in your heart.

Breathe slowly and deeply, allowing all stress to unwind from your body and mind. Let go of any worries, concerns, and anxieties from the day, as you move into the *feeling* awareness of your body. Feel your breath, your heartbeat, and all the sensations within your body, realizing that every exhale serves to take you deeper into your true essence.

Once you both begin to feel comfortable and connected, move to the next step.

❧ Step Two

Come into a yab-yum position. This is where the woman sits on top of the man and wraps her legs around the back of his body. Hold one another in love as you come to a face-to-face position.

Close your eyes and begin to call down your soul's essence into the chamber of your mouth. Tune in to the spiritual aspects of your being and qualities of the soul family and lineage that you belong to. Feel their support and presence surrounding you as you receive the codes and unique frequencies of your soul.

Use the breath to draw these energies into your mouth. When I did this, I saw with my inner eyes Aramaic words and symbols written in a light language on the inside of my mouth. The more consciously I inhaled and exhaled, the brighter these words shone.

When both partners feel truly connected to the soul, and they feel its presence pulsating in their mouths, move to the next step.

❧ Step Three

Hold one another as if you were about to kiss, and bring your mouths close, leaving a gap wide enough to breathe (see page 110).

The man inhales through his mouth, and gently, deliberately exhales into the woman's mouth.

She receives his breath through her open mouth and guides it deep into her being. She consciously *feels* the essence of her beloved—his heart, his soul, his longings, his dreams, his prayers, his light, and *all* that he is. She feels his breath pass through her throat, into her lungs and heart. She allows it to move into the mystical inner worlds of love, light, truth, and expansion.

From this place the woman sends her energy up, gathering together her light, her love, her heart, her soul, her longings, her dreams, her prayers, and *all* that she is. She pulls this essence from the very depths of her being, while remaining connected with the man's soul essence that has gathered in her mouth. Then she merges the two and exhales deliberately, lovingly, and gently into his mouth as he takes this breath into him.

This is the secret teaching. You have to merge the very depths of matter with the finest frequencies of light. The "matter" is your physical body, the history of this life and all others, the personality, the enduring principle—the heart and guts of your character—the rich, embodied human being. The "light" is your untouched, radiant, pure soul. It is the elegant, gentle sweetness of your purity, your true self—unprotected, innocent, and free.

In your mouths, as you share the nashakh, matter and light meet, merge, and marry. With that awareness, pass your holy breath into your partner, knowing that when your partner breathes out into you, the very same thing is passed back to you. This is not just ordinary breath that you are passing one another, but spirit. Let us remind ourselves again, that *spirit* and *breath* have the same meaning in many of the ancient languages.

With that knowledge, continue to share breath for as long as feels comfortable.

This divine kiss can also merge into circular breathing. But don't get tangled in mental definitions.

As you drop into a natural rhythm, let go of any technique and allow yourself to surrender deeply to the mystery. Use this time to pray, to merge, and to experience union. Allow all resistances to melt and blur into the light of your love. Let it penetrate and surround you.

Pray for God's love to unite you, to bless you, to comfort you, and to nurture you. Ask to experience the deeper forms of union—the mystical, unteachable, and unspeakable realms of bliss and innocence. Know that they will carve so deeply into your being that nothing will ever be the same again. Amen.

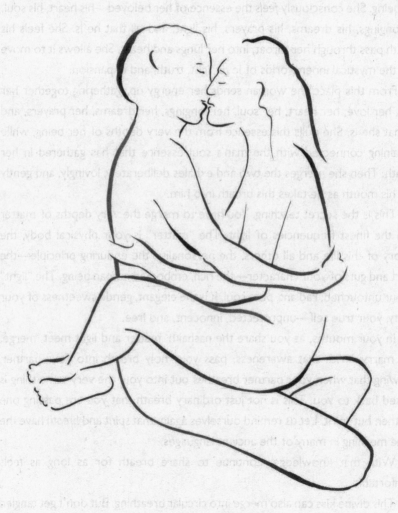

Nashakh, the divine kiss

DRIVE

Drive—to propel oneself and others in a specified direction

Love without power dissolves into an astral, weak fairy tale. Love without strength crumbles into an ungrounded, chaotic mess. Power without love becomes a game of control, fear, and tyranny. Discipline without joy becomes an intense, self-defeating, oppressive hell.

These polarities of power and compassion, surrender and will, direct penetration and gentle opening, fire and water, can all merge into one seamless flow. Each quality is used at different times to create the most appropriate change.

One reason why so few people have reached awakening is that they have taken one or the other path and not included both. Many beings are scared to shine their full light and power, too afraid to stand out. With drive, anything that stands in the way of your growth is dealt with swiftly: any attachment, any fear, any emotion, any person of any sort that hinders or distracts from your goal is healed, released, or removed. Drive cuts through any and all illusions and ignorance to awaken the soul. It is death to the masks of the wounded self and surrender in action to self and the beloved.

Drive is unmoved by worldly troubles, cares, or concerns. It is direct, clear movement that dissolves obstacles in its way, cutting through the tap roots of egoism, no matter how its actions are perceived by others. It is compassion for the soul and the bigger picture; it is not stopped by the protestations of society, parents, friends, or the wounded self. It is personal power harnessed to divine will. Once truly ignited it can never be stopped until all obstacles and ignorance are destroyed.

Enlightenment is a process of destruction.

ADYASHANTI

Drive provides rapidly accelerated evolution—where no stone is left unturned—and is for those that wish to be fully enlightened, no matter what. With drive, one is ready and willing to do absolutely anything to awaken. Drive involves accepting what you need to grow, rather than what you want. Comfort and fitting in to our wound-driven society are low on the list of priorities for those with drive. For this reason the actions of drive are often not appreciated until well after it has been received and can initially be greeted by the wounded self with judgment, resentment, and anger.

The heart of drive is the heart of spaciousness, which allows others to be in their pain and suffering so they may grow. It is relentless in that it is not stopped by pain or suffering; it feels all without hiding, flinching, or avoiding. This is the heart of acceptance, accepting what must be for the highest good.

Drive requires great passion, inner balance, dedication, and wisdom to flow with it and implement its actions and directions. Wisdom here is the ability to see beyond appearances to the true clinging, suffering, and need of a person. Acting on this directly arises from being objective, calm, and clear in understanding how and why the wounded self protects, hides, and cloaks itself.

Drive is a way of being that arises when one is fully dedicated to self and God. It is uncompromising, direct, and unflinching. Drive is action orientated. It does, not thinks about doing, or talks about doing. It is love made manifest through action. Holy desire is the engine of your car; drive is the four wheels of your car. Drive is courage *in the world* and is the external application of holy desire. Drive collects all the pieces of yourself that you need to get to what, whom, and where you desire to be, to become, and to go.

Paradoxically drive becomes a process of surrender that grinds down anything that stands in the way between your pure soul and your wounded or lower self. This leads to total harmlessness, as no reaction, no harm, can affect you when you have no harm, no violence, no triggers left within you. Then these forces can be wielded in order to serve love effectively, as and when required.

Sometimes the bludgeon is required. The bludgeon that cuts to the bone, that illumines illusion in the most direct and uncompromising manner. My Friends, do not compromise with the illusion in yourself and others. Be radically honest, for this serves love. Be frank, be directly engaging, and do not shirk your responsibility toward the growth of your soul.

Drive leads people into the dark night of the soul. Drive builds up people's characters and dissolves their small selves, to lead them into an awakening that will have true impact as it is based on authentic, deep, lived experiences of the darkest places a human being can go. Once you have lived through this experience, then anything is possible for you. You have reclaimed your power from the darkness and can now wield it yourself.

Drive forges the soul into a diamond, by burning the dross away, leaving only that which is immortal. The doubts, the voices, the trials, and the tribulations are all voices of the tempter that does not wish you to stand in your power, in the truth. Here there is no "your" truth or "my" truth; there is only one truth that we both align to.

Holy Prayer

━━━━━━━━━━━━━━━━✦━━━━━━━━━━━━━━━━

Beloved Father Mother God, please help me find the drive within myself to conquer all my obstacles. Help me find my inner power and blast my way through my illusions in to You. Help me to align with my drive and serve only the fulfillment of that expression. Align my drive with self-love and integrity, serving the fullness of my soul. Amen.

♫ Sacred Action

What do you really desire and want? What is stopping you from doing this? What excuses do you tell yourself that stop you from being full blooded, action orientated, passionate, and direct in achieving your heart's desires? Name five of them.

Then take a moment to consider the following questions. Are you lazy? Why? Would you rather live a second-rate life than live the life of your dreams? Why? Do you need to be more physical in your life? Are you doing a job that is your passion? Are you doing a job that will directly lead you into eternity and the embrace of the beloved? Why not?

Below are some questions to help you stop thinking and start *doing*. Use the questions above to think about what you might start doing, and then write down your answers to each questions below. And then get to action right away!

- When you think of [topic], what are you most excited about?
- How does this [topic] fit in with your vision of your highest self?
- What is your goal in this area? Now double it. What is the version of the goal that is so big you are afraid to admit (even to yourself) for fear of failure?
- What's holding you back?
- What support do you need to move forward?
- What one next step would make the biggest impact to move you forward?
- What would achieving this bring you?
- Close your eyes and ask each major decision making system for advice: What does your head say? What does your heart say? What does your gut say? How can you reconcile the three?
- Dig even deeper. What do you really want?
- What are you waiting for?
- What *were* you afraid of?

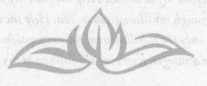

FAITH

Faith—complete trust or confidence in someone or something, especially in times of unknowing or uncertainty

If you want to strengthen your faith, you will need to soften inside. For your faith to be rock solid, your heart needs to be soft as a feather.

ELIF SHAFAK, *THE FORTY RULES OF LOVE:*
A NOVEL OF RUMI

And all the opposites of the universe are present within each and every one of us. Therefore the believer needs to meet the unbeliever residing within. And the nonbeliever should get to know the silent faithful in him. Until the day when one reaches the stage of Insan-I Kâmil, the perfect human being, faith is a gradual process and one that necessitates its seeming opposite: disbelief.

ELIF SHAFAK, *THE FORTY RULES OF LOVE:*
A NOVEL OF RUMI

Faith arises from the direct experience of love many times over until you no longer believe in it, but *know* it. The more direct experiences of love we have, the more faith we have in it. Faith is not sitting around with a wish to have faith. Faith is active. You put divine will into action; you do what you can and trust the next steps will happen through grace unfolding, because you have put the effort in to make it happen.

Belief may arise from a conviction of the mind, but faith never can. Its place of being is in the soul, and no one can possess it unless his soul is awakened by the inflowing of Love. So that, when we pray to the Father to increase our faith it is a prayer for the increase of Love. Faith is based on the possession of this Love.

FROM CHRIST YESHUA'S TEACHINGS AS
REVEALED BY JAMES E. PADGETT IN
DIVINE LOVE: TRANSFORMING THE SOUL

Faith is fidelity to the truth. It stays with the truth when all else comes crashing down. It always follows your highest potential. Faith is something you know in the core of your being, something you can always rely on. It is staying constant in the truth, despite any and all circumstances.

You place your faith and loyalty in what you choose to value. If it is a temporary person or belief of this world, then the loyalty will always be *of* the temporary, of this world. It can crumble. True faith can only serve one master. If you place your loyalty in what is eternal, then so shall it be. If you are loyal to love, loyal to God, then it is love and God you shall receive and become.

To be vigilant in every moment, to value and be loyal to love in every situation, is the work. It is only when we withdraw love from any relating or situation that thoughts and emotions of separation arise. As these emotions arise, ask what you are being loyal to.

Trust the infinite love that is creating you moment by moment. In this you trust that whatever people, books, lessons, and events cross your path are in your highest interests for growth, leading you toward your highest potential. Every time you choose faith, you choose to be loyal to love.

True faith is the lived experience, the deep trust that gives us the strength to continue, to go forward, and to keep working on ourselves, because we know what we are working for is real. We become certain from our direct experience that love is real. This serves to take you further into the unknown, deepening your willingness and courage to go there.

To have faith means that we feel safe and secure in our essence and in God. We know that we are loved, that we love, and that we trust this flow in our lives. This flow is always there, ever present as our support, our ground, constant and reliable, even when we forget it or push it aside. The truth is, faith only seems to come and go. What really does come and go is the idea of *you*. You, rather than faith, come and go from your perception of life. It is the idea of you that stands in the way of faith manifesting fully in your life as true strength, stability, and eternal support.

When we have integrated faith's transformation into our lives, when our heart knows that God and love are real, when we are in harmony with this way of living and the choices we make in what to be loyal to, then we experience true strength. This strength does not waver, as it is based in the eternal, whereas our faith in another person, teacher, or teaching can change over time, for perceptions change as growth deepens. Evolving becomes quicker once we have true strength, as it leads us into deeper experience. In this true strength we experience life as wondrous and spontaneous, allowing it to unfold naturally. If we knew everything that was going to happen, there would be no real fun. Life would be boring! Faith allows existence to continually weave its magic, bringing more love into our lives and taking us ever deeper into previously unimagined possibilities.

As you travel the path, faith sustains, supports, and gives you solid ground. In true faith your life can change direction. Faith is giving yourself to life fully. As you evolve, faith deepens and changes its nature until the soul surrenders to God, which then becomes the support and ground for you. God herself holds and supports you. The ground that gives rise to you is also the ground and support to all life. When one experiences this—that the faith that is our support is the support of all beings also—one opens the doorway to soul realization: I Am.

Holy Prayer*

✦

Beloved Father Mother God, please help me to have more faith—such faith that will cause me to realize that I am Your divine angel, at one with You in very substance, not in image only. You are my beloved, Father Mother God, bestower of every good and perfect gift in my life. Only I, myself, can prevent Your divine love from changing me from the mortal to the immortal. Amen.

❧ Sacred Action

Do you have faith in yourself? Do you have faith in God? Do you have faith in anyone? Name three people you have faith in.

Why do you not have faith in yourself, God, or others? What incidents have happened in your life that made you distrust others, yourself, or God? What emotions are still left lurking within you that stop you from having more faith? Do you trust the flow of life and what is presented to you?

When you are presented with a choice of two actions, avenues, or opportunities, identify which one leads to more love, despite the material attractions presented. The more we feel love within us, the more we can trust

---

*This prayer was adapted from Christ Yeshua's teachings as revealed by James E. Padgett in *The Padgett Messages.*

ourselves in all situations. When we feel this love within ourselves, we have the ultimate reference point. Then we can ask the question: what is it I do not trust? Is it something within me I do not trust, or something in the other person or situation or opportunity I do not trust?

Faith is within. In your times of desperation and doubt, fear, and cynicism, ask: what would love do now?

Faith is not necessary when you know how things are going to work out— that is knowledge. However, in times of unknowing, faith sees you through to the other side. Faith is what gives you strength. Faith is that light in your heart that keeps on shining, even when all outside is darkness. Now is the time to keep that faith alive!

What do you require faith in *now?* In this moment can you breathe *complete* trust into your experience? Allow yourself to fill with this faith, trusting ever deeper, beyond anything you have ever known.

This is your quest, Beloved One; for the next eleven days, have full and complete faith. Breathe through all doubts, all divisions, and all distractions. Focus only on your faith, and allow yourself the experience of knowing fully and completely the power of such a force.

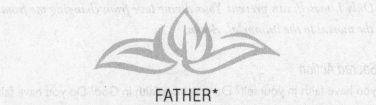

FATHER*

Father—a man's essence in relation to his child, his creations, and the origin of all his creative expressions

The masculine aspect of father is the seed origin in the early history of a child, a creative project, a company, and all our intimate relationships. A father gives care, strength, and protection to allow all these to grow.

---

*This pearl, which is mainly directed toward men, is parallel to the Mother pearl (page 39), which is mainly directed toward women. Of course everyone can gain from reading and absorbing the importance of both pearls for the masculine and feminine essences inside all of us.

A father gives an emotional imprint to his children that allows them to become who they really are as unique individuals.

Becoming a father is an important rite of passage for a man. It brings him deeper into his pure masculine essence and further embodies his soul. It balances him into wholeness through a mixture of tenderness, strength, care, and deep presence. Unfortunately many fathers never complete the true initiation of fatherhood. In our divine design we are meant to complete this initiation over a three-year period, from conception to when the child is two years old.

To be a father requires constant presence from the heart, loving consistently and persistently. The other needs love and responds most to love. As a man grows into fatherhood, his healing edges and wounds arise through his interactions with his children and his partner. They show him where he still needs to heal. He, in turn, provides them with the safety, security, reassurance, and modeled strength from the heart and hara that become the basis of his masculine side. Parenting is a two way street: giving and receiving love in all the ways we need and deserve it.

The father quality is important to have integrated in intimate relationships for both men and women as it allows them to rest, accept, and feel safe in their magnetic foundation, sexuality, and womb/hara. This allows them both to feel and express their depths. The integrated and healed father quality is innate in all men and is activated through conscious birthing and healing the wounds of your childhood associated with your own father.

This integrated father quality provides a pillar that allows relationships to work because there is a still, unshakable core that cares for and looks after both people. In tantra, Shakti is seen as constantly dancing around the still, calm masculine, sitting in perfect balance and equipoise. When the man is this, Shakti can play, weave, and create to her heart's content.

The dance of intimate relating involves many roles. At certain times we all need to be a father- or mother-type figure to our inner child and our partner to allow deeper emotional openings and expression to happen. This does not mean you become their literal father or mother, merely the archetypal role for a moment or two.

Becoming a father means you have to let go of your old identity and change yourself. You die to part of your old self to become more selfless, more patient, more giving. You let go of your old self-centered life for another life. A gentle flame of love ignites in your heart, a flame that is perpetual: it is always there. A chamber of your heart opens up. True love for your children is felt from the same place where a father prays to God: the core of your soul. A human father would sacrifice his life in a heartbeat for his children. He would do anything and give up anything to protect his children.

A father has the strength to say no, to create boundaries that will in fact free his partner and children to be who they really are. He allows everyone within his care to become exactly what they are supposed to be; he allows and brings forth their individual essences and deepest qualities, affording them the field, the space, and the ground for them to be and bloom.

Just so, a father of an idea, a project, or company will also allow his "children" to grow into what they are designed to be innately. A father brings forth the divine blueprint of all he is entrusted with by allowing, guiding, and supporting. His familiar resonance is a comforting beacon inviting his partner, children, and ideas more into the world of form: into embodiment. This union of masculine and feminine creates a gateway, a portal, through which more of the soul can express in the world.

The following are aspects of the father's soul role.

- To be an emotionally clear, calm, reassuring strength and pillar of the masculine
- To engender and deepen trust and respect through his own integrity, right guidance, and actions
- To withstand and process adversity in the whirlwind of emotions
- To share the loving, strong, gentle, and vulnerable masculine
- To create a degree of discipline and healthy emotional boundaries for all
- To encourage the remembrance of soul presence
- To remember his own soul agreement with his partner and chil-

dren, and why they have chosen each other, what they need to learn from and with each other

♦ To help create a safe, strong, emotional, and spiritual container for physical and soulful growth within a Sacred Relationship

Holy Prayer

Beloved Father Mother God, please help me become the true father within me. Spark this remembrance within me! Help me feel and release my pain, sadness, lack of trust, and hurt with my own father. Beloved Father God, I feel You are my real, true, and beautiful Father. I know You are always here for me, always ready to take me into Your loving arms. Help me be here for my partner and children. Amen.

⚡ Sacred Action

Connect to your breath and ask yourself the following questions, writing down the answers. Do you feel the need to control your partner at times? Do you trust your intuition? Do you feel unresolved anger or frustration with your father? Do you provide all that you need? Do you take time to truly process your emotions? Do you feel resistance to your partner's emotions? Where does your guidance come from? Can you express the truth even if it is hard for others to hear? Do you have clear boundaries in your relationships? Can you draw strong boundaries for your child and partner even if it means turning loved ones away? Do you exercise authority in your life and your relationships? Are you honest with yourself and your partner? Are you financially secure and established?

Then connect to your breath again as you ask yourself these questions concerning your own father, writing down your answers: Did your father have strong boundaries? Did your father try to control your mother? Did your father trust his own and your mothers' intuitions? Did your father provide all that you needed? Did your father show and process all his emotions? Did your father show resistance to others' emotions? Did your father express the truth? Did your father exercise authority? Was your father honest? Was your father financially secure and established?

Read over your answers, bringing awareness and breath to your responses. Take your time as you come to terms with what you have written.

FEARLESS

Fearless—embodying courage, cool calm awareness, and an absence of fear and unconsciousness

FEAR: Fear Expects A Reaction
FEAR: False Evidence Appears Real
FEAR: Feeling Emotion And Refusing
FEAR: Forgetting Expecting Analyzing Refuting
FEAR: Forget Everything And Run

The mind of fear collates all kinds of evidence from every possible imaginable source to substantiate its fear, making it real. The mind of fear does not want to feel any deeper to the source of its fear, preferring to stay in the reactive charge. Fear is forgetfulness of our innate love and forgiveness and seeks out others to follow its agenda. Fear sees itself as a great protector of our souls, when in fact fear is the protector of the deeper emotions found within our wounded selves. When felt, fear is a sign that something far deeper is happening, waiting for us to investigate it.

Love holds no fear in it; perfect love casts out all fear. There are quite simple things you can do to see for yourself whether you are in love or fear. Many of us tend to spiritualize or bypass our fears, making them an intellectual exercise with imagined scenarios, visualizations, or affirmations to help placate our fears temporarily. This is all bypassing a simple truth: if you are scared of something, you have not brought love to it. So do the most fearful thing you can imagine. For example, if you are scared of deep water, learn scuba diving. Scared of heights? Learn skydiving. Scared of spiders? Go to a forest full of them. Scared of intimacy in a relationship? Time to bare your soul. Scared of living alone? Spend a month camping in Nature. Scared of losing your job? Take a sabbatical. Scared of having no money? Go and live for a month with no money and go begging.

Feel the fear; feel the inevitable emotions that arise from these activities. You will learn more about yourself and conquer the fear faster through this activity than through a month of meditating. Standing up to your fear comes from manifesting your passion for growth, your passion to become love put into solid, grounded action!

The fears held in the mind can work out through your body and vice versa. For example, wounds in the emotional body can pop up viscerally through the physical body in aches, strains, and pains. Fear is felt in the body-mind. Breath becomes short, sharp, ragged, and fast. Hormones of adrenaline fire as the fight-or-flight response kicks in. The survival instincts of the body, survival instincts of the wound, survival instincts of the splintered mind will all struggle and fight to stay alive. Everything in Nature wants to survive. Fear contracts us and wants to survive. That is its nature.

When you are centered in your soul, you are able to react to fear differently. You may have a life-threatening situation to your body-mind, yet you yourself feel nothing emotionally because you have healed the fear within you. You witness the scenario playing out and take calm action to help your body-mind survive. You are not run by the fear; you do not panic. Your soul is in charge, not the fear.

For example, I (Padma) did a nighttime scuba dive half a mile out in the Pacific Ocean. As I descended into the black water abyss, miles deep, my body-mind instinctively reacted, firing the fight-or-flight mechanism. It wanted to panic. I observed this strong reaction in my body, calmly arose to the surface, and breathed deeply. Within five minutes I descended back again into the black underwater world to enjoy my amazing dive.

Fear plays itself out in all kinds of relationships. Fear of being seen, fear of being abandoned, fear of being hurt, fear of not being good enough, fear that manifests in fight or flight (arguments and storming away). Fear always lies on the surface of your emotions and, in truth, is a welcoming sign that a series of deeper emotions lie underneath, waiting for your attention and embrace to feel and release them. Fear of being seen can be shame for how bad you feel inside. Fear of being abandoned (or abandoning another) may come from your parents having abandoned you when you were young. Fear of being hurt may be activating a deep wound within you. Fear of not being good enough for your partner stems from feelings of unworthiness, possibly from your ancestral line.

Fearlessness comes with the courage to feel the fear and dive into it, to have an attitude of innocent curiosity and investigation, to embrace part of yourself that feels left out, isolated, hurt, betrayed, or denied. Fearless beings have delved into the deepest parts of themselves, alone and with others, and confronted their shadow. They have brought the shadow out in front of them to see it fully, rather than have it lie untended to in the background. They have the courage to go where they have never gone before. They want to bring love into every part of themselves and feel the truth.

The old paradigm is based on fear. The new paradigm is based on love. Both cannot exist together. As we transition together from the old into the new, let us be tender to ourselves. Let us be brave and dive deep. Let us find our core, our strength, and may we dismantle all the old structures we have created that keep us in fear. Love needs no protection. Love can never be harmed.

Holy Prayer

✦

Beloved Father Mother God, please help me feel my fears. Please show me, in my life this very week, all my fears. Help me have the courage to dive into them. Help me feel the deeper emotions that lie underneath my fears, and help me release them. Give me the strength and courage to stand strong and to fearlessly embrace the parts of me that need love. Please send me Your divine love. Amen.

◈ Sacred Action

Beloved One, what are you most afraid of in this moment? You have turned to this Pearl of Wisdom for a reason—can you identify what you are most scared of? Who are you most scared of? Why? What emotions lie underneath these fears?

Can you befriend your fear? Can you move closer to it in prayer and meditation and hold its substance in your heart? That is the work my friend: to parent your fear, taking it as your own child and offering it your mature, wise, and living presence.

Now go *do* one simple thing that you have been afraid to do in the past.

Now go *say* one simple thing that you have been afraid to speak of in the past.

Keep it simple and parent your fearful child through it. Go skinny-dipping, walk naked in the moonlight, try a new food, take a samba class, write a poem, climb a tree, or introduce yourself to a stranger who catches your attention—the list is endless; you know what to do.

Stay calm, keep breathing, and make it fun! This is a new moment, and you are filled with the presence of love! Let it cast out fear.

FREEDOM

Freedom—the state of feeling open, expansive, and able to act, speak, feel, or think in alignment with the truth of your being

In true freedom possessiveness is impossible, any form of control incomprehensible, any attempt at manipulation laughable. Respect for the sovereignty of yourself and another as a human and divine being allows us to deeply experience *all* things without expectation or need. Ultimately through this respect, along with prayer and healing of wounds, we become free. We are connected to love as our Source, and holy revelations open up to reveal the full power of this freely embodied love.

Holy Tantra can correct the addiction we have to the transcendent as well as the attachment we may have to the body. Sacred Relationship has the power to fuse all pairs of opposites into union within a harmonious energy field. By bringing both the transcendent urge and juiciness of life together, we fuse the fullness of our divinity with our humanity—and that, my Beloved Friend, is freedom. This is the vision we can strive to serve. We must treasure this urge and this longing within us. The old paradigm may rear its fearsome head in a last attempt to fully claim us—and that is where we have to help one another out. Let us remember to act with kindness, consciousness, and patience.

> *We must be willing to get rid of*
> *the life we've planned, so as to have*
> *the life that is waiting for us.*
>
> *The old skin has to be shed*
> *before the new one can come.*
>
> *If we fix on the old, we get stuck.*
> *When we hang onto any form,*
> *we are in danger of putrefaction.*
>
> *Hell is life drying up.*
>
> JOSEPH CAMPBELL,
> *A JOSEPH CAMPBELL COMPANION:*
> *REFLECTIONS ON THE ART OF LIVING*

As we grunt and groan our way through the birthing pains of the new paradigm, releasing supposed forms of comfort, security, and safety, we realize in actual fact that they offered us none of those things at all. The old paradigm's trick is to keep us stuck in a nongrowth situation. It has encouraged us to seek authority outside of ourselves, to strive to "make it" in the system, to limit our horizons, and to stay locked down in relationships, jobs, circumstances, and states of health that are depleting, deadening, and destructive. Take a look at some of the internal differences between living in the old paradigm and living in the new paradigm.

Old paradigm—you are constantly seeking freedom and it irritates you if you don't feel it; you run from pain, you create conflict, you blame others, and you withdraw your love

New paradigm—you feel free within and connected to the quantum field of all possibilities; in your life—and all your relationships—you continually seek to expand your horizons, both inner and outer; you embrace discomfort with trust; you have harmonious intentions; you are responsible for your thoughts and actions; and you pray like mad to continue loving

Freedom requires boundaries, paradoxically. Freedom is the willing capacity to discover more of who you are. Freedom blooms when you have healed all the hurts of incarnation and stand in your pure soul. Freedom awakens when you fulfill your soul's desires to their utmost and live this. Perhaps the greatest freedom is being exactly who you are and expressing this without reservation, hesitation, or delay, in all ways, physically, emotionally, mentally, soulfully, and sexually.

Freedom ripens when you are honestly and totally content to be alone, all-one, in all ways. Freedom is consecrated when God is your partner and you are worthy enough to accept this humbly and confidently. Freedom binds no one and frees everyone to be whatever they wish to be. Freedom is when love is the whole of the law you live by, and in this understanding you can do what you want.

Freedom is *not* hedonism, doing whatever your wounded selfish self wants, doing whatever your hurt inner child screams for, and causing harm to others. It is grounded in an experience of the vastness of being, a knowing of your true self, which is eternal. When we live our commitment to true freedom, everything—yes, *everything*—serves and sustains who we really are and who we are becoming.

Holy Prayer

Beloved Father Mother God, help me to free myself (and my partner) from the old paradigm with its myriad of false promises and painful shackles. Help me to be brave enough to see all of my possessiveness, ways of controlling, and attempts at manipulation. I do not want to play with these self-generated powers—for they are not powers at all, merely traps. Traps that I alone place myself in. I desire to be a free being, and to expand that blessing to my partner and to all beings in my life. Freedom is Your gift of love to us, and I desire to love in that way. Help me to become aware of how I may embody this prayer and to gently realign me with Your comforting grace and wisdom. Amen.

§ *Sacred Action*

Beloved One, take a moment to consider where you are *not* free in your life. How are you going to change that? What step are you going to take right *now* that will make you freer?

Freedom is a step-by-step process and journey. Each step taken, however small, gives a signal to life and to God that you are ready and willing. Then the next step will be shown to you. We are all free to choose any action, whether it be loving or unloving. What choices have you made today that are loving, or unloving? How could you be more free in your body, your emotions, your expression, your sexual movements, and your soul?

Write down three things for each quality.

In the spirit of living in true freedom, read, integrate, and embody these fifteen principles of new-paradigm relating.

- Happiness is irrelevant—be free to embody your courageous self
- Your only question should be—am I growing?
- Your wounded feelings are your responsibility
- You are never upset for the reasons you think you are
- You do not have or strive for control over another
- There is 100 percent conscious awareness and loving contribution from both people in your relationship
- There is balance between physical, sexual, emotional, psychological, and soulful stimulation and relaxation
- You have transparent communication: no secrets, lies, or half-truths
- You make requests, never demands
- You make your partner more important than your past
- You are free; your partner is free
- You are trustworthy; your partner is trustworthy
- You have taken a quantum step beyond the ancestral wounding in relationship
- You never repeat your parents' shortcomings
- You always hang in there; if your partner is just as committed, it will pass

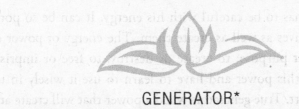

GENERATOR*

Generator—a dynamic, action-orientated being that creates, orchestrates, or manifests something

Generating and catalyzing yourself and others are part of the expression of masculine power. The generator provides a spark of light, a spark of excitement and adventure—the power of Ra. Ra catalyzes all who come around him, giving them inspiration, motivation, a spark, a push, a nudge deeper into themselves. A true generator does not care what people think of him; he is a pioneer, breaking down barriers, catalyzing growth, bringing people more into themselves by illuminating and dissolving shields and walls.

A generator is fun, exciting, and sometimes challenging to be around. The pace of life he creates is hard for many to keep up with. Relentlessly creative, bursting with ideas that he manifests into form, he is an adventurer, willing to go where few dare to tread. He lives life out of the box, and is wildly spontaneous, creating transformation wherever he goes. He liberates stuck energy in order to create. He manifests with grace and ease.

A generator has the spark of life liberated within him. Once this spark is freed, it must create, or it will burn him up. This spark creates and needs fuel to create, for this is its purpose. This fuel can be the energies of the wounded self, in which case he will create unloving but seemingly fun and exciting projects. Or the fuel can be the soul, in which case he will create projects that bring more love, consciousness, and dynamic experiences for others.

---

*This pearl, which is mainly directed toward men, is parallel to the Womb pearl (page 88), which is mainly directed toward women. Of course everyone can gain from reading and absorbing the importance of both pearls for the masculine and feminine essences inside all of us.

A generator has to be careful with his energy. It can be so potent that it can ruin lives as well as create them. The energy of power can be used for either purpose: to create or destroy, to free or imprison. Generators have this power and have to learn to use it wisely in tandem with the heart. True generators wield a power that will create at all times. It is their nature to never let up, never give in, never stop until what they are doing has manifested into form. This is a vital part of the creation process: every undertaking needs a generator otherwise nothing will be manifested.

Spiritually speaking, generators who are teachers are inexhaustible in their service. They keep on creating and creating. If they are unbalanced, they can get lost in this process, doing themselves, their bodies, and others harm. As a transformative force, they will keep working on their students with inspiration, motivation, and ruthless compassion until a breakdown, and breakthrough, is made. This unstoppable primal force lies deep within us all. Teeming with life and passion, this force can be as scary and threatening as it is inspiring and exciting. When we encounter such power, people can become fully motivated and totally inspired to make radical changes in their lives or become scared that they will become annihilated, lost in this vortex.

There are no taboos, no conventions ruling a true generator. They are here to create and make something new when their power is harnessed to the soul and God. The generator can create light. The testes are the biological light generators of the male body, like the ovaries are for the feminine. Testes are the essence of masculinity, giving vitality, joyful exuberance, power, and life force. On a deeper level they anchor a soft, deep, loving male essence. They help fuel honor when united with the heart.

The testes hold the energy of the heart in manifestation, and they serve to embody and transmit the pure male principle of creation here in the body. When a man is deeply embodied in his testes, his power and presence are deeply felt. In Sacred Relationship this allows both man and woman to relax and surrender more deeply into their container.

Holy Prayer

✦

Beloved Father Mother God, please help me generate more energy through my testes. I want to be powerful, generating, and electrifying. Please help me feel and release my unworthiness; emotions of rejection, hatred, anger, and resentment toward the feminine; all past pains with my father and my sexual partners; grief; and sadness. Allow me to find balance with the feminine. Help me to take rest and relaxation. Beloved God, keep my creations pure and holy. Guide my creations in accordance with holy desire and impeccable integrity. Amen.

✜ *Sacred Action*

Inhale glowing, iridescent, deep wine red energy down into the seed of your testes; then slowly exhale out. Repeat this six times.

Inhale radiant, glowing, iridescent, fluid white energy deep into the seed of your testes; then slowly exhale out. Repeat this six times.

Inhale shining, glowing, iridescent fluid black energy deeply into the seed of your testes; then slowly exhale out. Repeat this six times.

Breathe these cycles of deep wine red, radiant white, and shining black twice more.

GIVING

Giving—providing love, emotional support, time, and presence

To truly give is to receive, and it always leads to more joy. Giving is an extension of the love you feel within you, and it is a natural effect of its cause: love. It is not an obligation or duty, a rule or dogma. Many people believe giving is the cause, not the effect, but it is the effect of your healing and wholeness. It flows naturally and spontaneously in all situations; it does not need a reason.

Many believe that giving can alleviate their karma, that by doing good works they are clearing their karmas and their soul wounds. This is not true. People still must do their inner work and healing, and once they do, they have more to give, from a sincere and spontaneous place within them.

When you feel love, giving will naturally and effortlessly extend itself. Giving selflessly, without expectation of reward back, actually opens your heart a little bit more and opens the crown chakra channel to receive more from beloved God. Giving is a graceful flow from the heart that enjoys the love and wisdom bubbling forth and naturally wishes to share this with anyone and everyone in *any* situation. For when we feel more joy, more beauty, and more God from what we give out, all we want to do is share even more of it—and so the spiral rises ever higher.

Giving is shared with everyone on the level they can receive it. From the beggar in the street to the avid spiritual student, each soul requires something different in every different moment. The open heart knows what to give in every moment to any person, no matter where they are in the spirals of evolution. There is no greater joy than seeing another transform in front of you and feeling that peace and satisfaction within the shared heart.

When you are living from your deepest self, giving is what you do in every situation. You have unlimited energy to do so as this energy stems from God, and God is never on holiday. Time becomes more important as you choose not to waste it. Instead you maximize time in order to be an open vessel for the sharing and extending of transformation. Those who live in the highest spheres of service in the world are constantly serving others and have little time for anything else, save their own meditations of course!

It is here that the very word *service* becomes a misnomer. Service is our most natural, effortless way of being. It is the result of the very flow of life itself. And when we are in this flow, selfishness and hoarding become drains and blocks to your full expression, contracted, fearful, and heavy. In true giving, you no longer keep much of anything for yourself as there is the recognition that there is no separate self to keep anything for.

Of course, the more we heal ourselves, the less of a separate self there will be. If you think you are giving and you are not enjoying it, then it is not true giving. Giving is never a burden; it is lightness. Service is never a duty; it is a voluntary willingness. Service includes all of yourself in it, and does not leave anything out. Service is not something to do. It is a way of life, a way of being. It is God's lifestyle.

Giving is our nature. It's how life itself operates through the sacred hoop, the circuit of life that flows into us and out through us, back into the universe. If we block this circuit of life and love, we start to stagnate. Giving continually realigns us to the constant flow of change, growth, and newness that is life. To tune in to life, tune in to giving; to tune in to what your service is, tune in to the life force. Then you will be guided on the most magical journey back to your true, joyful self in harmony with the rhythms of life. Just as atoms whirl around each other in harmony, keeping each other in existence through their whirling, simply being what they are created to be, so can we realign ourselves. Through giving, we align with the way that we have been created to be—the way that gives us the most joy. Giving is our completion into love.

Try it now; give to a stranger today, even if it is only a smile. Take the initiative in giving. Do not wait to be asked, but do whatever is needed. Give to yourself also. Set times to meditate, to enjoy life, to have a holiday, to appreciate the beauty around you. Have alone time away from all others, and do not neglect it. You are as important as that meeting, that client, your family, or even helping others get their needs met. You have to give yourself the time to be *not of the world*. To maintain this balance is to maintain inner harmony, and this opens the gates to more love and peace flowing through you. Taking one step toward God means God is given permission to take ten steps toward you. To do this requires periods of giving to yourself in retreat and meditation, so that when you return to the active life serving others, you have stabilized your own state of consciousness. Then, it is always available.

Holy Prayer

✦

Beloved Father Mother God, show me what I can give to others today. Show me what I can give to support another today. Help me release the fear and unworthiness that stops me from giving freely of myself to others. Help me share the love I feel in my alone moments with others—today and every day. Amen.

ᕳ *Sacred Action*

Go into a public park, get on a public bus or train, get out there in the world. Smile at people. Silently say from your heart *I love you*, to each soul you meet. What happens? How do you feel?

Beloved One, have you been hoarding yourself away? Have you been cutting yourself off from human and animal connection? Have you been holding back from yourself or from another that you know in your deepest heart truly *needs* something from you on this day? Come forward now, today, and allow yourself to share, to engage, and to exchange.

Ask yourself what you could give today, and then give it. Ask your heart how you may give to yourself and others, and then do it.

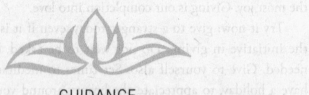

GUIDANCE

Guidance—clear and concise advice or information aimed at resolving a problem or difficulty, especially given by someone coming from a higher understanding

The masculine within us guides the feminine within us with clear and precise direction gleaned from a higher perspective and skilled navigating thresholds, while at the same time honoring the feminine's free will. The masculine (both within and externalized) must feel free to share his loving guidance if the feminine (within and externalized) is lost, unaware, or about to make an unloving or uninformed decision.

Guidance and decision making that affect a relationship have two potential avenues. Some direction and decision requires both the masculine and feminine aspects to be considered and consulted. Other times it is best to rely on the masculine aspect for the decision that is best for the relationship as a whole. For example, if a couple wishes to relocate to another country, mutual dialogue considering both masculine and feminine factors is best. Yet, in another example, if there is too much procrastination in staying in an unloving and no-growth environment, and both agree that this is so, yet the feminine partner or feminine part of the self is caught in her comfort zone, the masculine partner or masculine part of the self has to be firm, strong, and clear in making the decision.

Deciding, taking clear action, and moving the energy of a relationship forward are masculine qualities. While each soul has to follow its heart's desire, our free will is often clouded and subverted by our underlying emotional wounds, which often seek to hide in a false form of safety. Often we follow familiar patterns that are not the most loving avenue for us to grow in. Sometimes in cases such as these, tough decisions need to be made to honor the growth of a soul. Leaving behind old ways of being and the emotional cords and binding this entails can be hard, especially if we are unwilling to let go of the past. This is where the masculine part of us comes in, guiding us to see the goal and go for it. Since this part of us is more detached, it can see the bigger picture without obstacle or interference. In the overview of a situation—a relationship, a dynamic, or an emotional maelstrom—the masculine can give valuable guidance to the feminine.

The masculine consciousness penetrates by its very nature. It strikes to the heart of a matter and sees it for what it is. It cuts through the veils of emotion and thought to reach the cause of it all. This can be very direct in telling the other the best course of action or in breaking down armor, illusions, shells, and resistance. It can be indirect as well, asking questions and gently teasing forth responses that get to the heart of the matter. It can mean giving your partner certain tasks to do that facilitate his or her growth. Sometimes the guide simply is totally receptive and opens up a space for listening and expression, and through this the feminine can open to her own clarity and knowing.

When a woman or the feminine part of the self feels she cannot hide and is totally seen by her masculine partner or self, it makes her more vulnerable, yet it is also a relief to be seen without having to pretend to be something. She has no role to play; she can simply be as she is. This is very relaxing! Guidance is accepted when the feminine trusts the masculine in the self or in a partner and there is a strong container in place in the relationship. The masculine is a reliable pillar in all kinds of situations, and this support brings the feminine into gratitude and safety as well as more humility and reverence for the masculine. This guidance is deeply nourishing to the soul as the feminine feels some of the deeper yearnings and urges within being fully met.

Guidance is not judgmental and does not use past events or arguments to hurt or prove a point against the other as is common in old paradigm relationships. This unresolved resentment and bitterness is poison to any relating. Following healthy guidance opens both partners to a deeper trust in life and in God, for in Sacred Relationships both man and woman see each other as Divine in certain ways and at certain times.

Receiving guidance is an art in itself. The more humble and open one is to receiving guidance, the more one can hear it and put it into action in one's life. This does not mean giving your power away as it actually deeply empowers you to be more of who you are. Humility and sovereignty combine to open up a channel for the exact pieces of guidance to be realized.

Sacred Relationships must have no agenda except the freedom of self and other to grow into union with God. If there are any other unhealed agendas, guidance will be blocked and not received. A true guide is fluid and spontaneous in the moment and adept in feeling and sensing where others are emotionally and what is appropriate in the moment. Guidance is a vessel for truth to be shared. The less the masculine aspect of self identifies in being a guide, the better guide he can be. If the guide is simply flowing with and enjoying life and an occasion arises to spontaneously share, he or she will—without investing in the situation or the outcome. This can be hard for someone who is attached to being with his or her partner, yet is not looking out for the partner's best interests. Sacred Relating is based on treating the other as you would like to be treated and wishing total freedom, love, and growth for the other, even at your own expense and the fear of the demise of the relationship.

Being a guide is fulfilling, rewarding, and spontaneous, as the guide simply opens up to grace and the guidance flows through him or her. It is not personal: it is evolutionary.

Holy Prayer

✦

Beloved Father Mother God, grant me the humility to accept guidance from my internal masculine and the external masculine of my partner. Help me be sovereign in Your divine light. Beloved God, help me let go of my defenses and see You working through my partner. Help me to be radically honest. Help me to trust my partner's guidance and—if I feel my own guidance is greater than my partner's—grace me the decency to be transparent with my feelings and to choose a reflection of greater guidance that I can respect, honor, and surrender unto. Amen.

§ *Sacred Action*

Sit face to face with your partner. Pray to God for humility, clarity, and loving kindness. When you feel this flow, share three pieces of guidance with your partner. Then allow the other to share three pieces of guidance with you.

What happens? Can you allow this guidance in? Can you trust it?

Beloved One, if you feel your guidance is more accurate than your partner's, then why are you with him or her? For what purpose do you surrender? It is inevitable, Beloved One; there will come an age when the feminine will surrender to worldly guidance from the masculine, and the masculine will seek out the feminine primordial wisdom of the soul—and on that day we shall come to know Divine Marriage.

HONOR

Honor—deep love, high respect, and great esteem for self or another; the love that makes a human lay down his life for his friend

When you honor someone or something, you bring it to life. You validate it; you authenticate it; you make it whole. You allow it to be seen and recognized, and in so doing, you help it to bloom into its full nature. When you honor someone or something, you make it real through your heart. In this process you bring others into your heart—you make a place for them and enfold, embrace, and protect them in your heart.

Honor is an action. King Arthur and the Knights of the Round Table demonstrated honor through following the truths of freedom, equality, mutuality, living for a cause greater than their individual selves. They follow this passionately and without ceasing, no matter what the cost or inconvenience. These qualities are marks of a true knight and true honor.

Honor is one of the foundations for all true relationships. It is a grounding quality of love that never wavers and is felt deep in the noble heart. It is a quality full of integrity, loyalty, chivalry, masculine power, and gentle strength. Honorable people always attract other people, because of this quality.

Knights were sworn to defend the poor, the weak, the helpless, and those who could not help themselves. The noble heart of honor holds the grandest vision and the deepest ideals as truths—and lives them daily. This honorable heart lives in men and women who may suffer failure and ridicule for their ideals. They may have been told to compromise just to fit in to the world, but they will never stray from what they know to be honorable and true. An honorable man protects the feminine; he is her pillar of strength. This allows her to be soft, because her strength comes from her softness. This softness can endure for far longer periods of time than masculine power. In honoring and being naturally in awe of the gentle, sustaining strength of the feminine, honorable men and women can evolve and deepen into their true nature.

> *Honour is a dynamic, living energy field in itself. . . .*
> *Honour is the energy field of every single human being*
> *when they are living their individual truth. . . . In the*
> *field of Honour, all human beings become one. . . . To*
> *honour someone is to hold them to their highest frequency*
> *no matter what their current frequency may be.*
>
> RICHARD RUDD, *THE GENE KEYS*

Honor means keeping your word, because honor does not lie. Honor is truth. An honorable person:

- speaks the truth and faces any consequences
- stands up for an ideal, for truth, and for love
- would rather die than be dishonorable
- does not pretend to be something he or she is not
- never takes more than he or she has given in life
- never cheats on his or her partner in feeling, thought, word, or deed
- would never do anything to manipulate or break up a partnership and never covets anyone else's partner or possessions
- never lives life *in fear* of being right or wrong
- never discusses someone's secrets with another
- never makes promises he or she cannot keep
- never manipulates sex or love to get something
- supports his or her partner and family, through thick and thin
- never stays silent when truth needs to be spoken
- sees each task through to completion
- never acts in desperation and impatience
- never betrays himself or herself or others
- takes responsibility for his or her actions, feelings, and thoughts, never blaming or acting in arrogance
- is not self-absorbed and does not ignore the sufferings of others
- never keeps the credit, honor, glory, and power for himself or herself alone
- never denies his or her own desires and heartfelt passions
- places love, truth, and God before job, home, and possessions, and even before children, parents, partner, or friends
- never gives to get, out of fear, duty, or pressure, or because others have said that he or she *should*
- never depends on anyone or anything for love and nourishment and never bows down to anyone or anything out of fear

Holy Prayer

———————————✦———————————

Beloved Father Mother God, please help me become an honorable person. Help me keep my soul agreements with You and all others.

Help me live by my word. Help me feel and release my emotions of fear, my weakness, my anger, my cowardice. Beloved Mother Father God, help me be still and stable within myself. Help me find my center. Thank You. Amen.

§ **Sacred Action**

Read this Pearl of Wisdom again through new eyes. Where are you not doing these acts of honor? When was the last time you were not honorable? Why were you not honorable? What was the *real* emotion behind your excuse for not being honorable?

Now, apply these questions to each and every quality of honor in the list above. Is there a theme, mentally and emotionally? What do you need to do to become an honorable person and fulfill this true masculine aspect of yourself?

INTELLIGENCE

Intelligence—the ability to acquire and apply knowledge in the present moment; a rhythmic presence that is fluid, spontaneous, and not bound to any rules

To understand the true nature of intelligence, let us look at the four different stages of knowing: information, knowledge, wisdom, and perfect knowing. Information is inputted into your system from reading, listening, watching TV, or looking at something from a sensory viewpoint. Knowledge takes this information into the mind, where you begin to memorize and contemplate it. It is still outside of you, but you are absorbing it and ruminating on it; you are making deductions and assertions. This logical process includes learning, thinking, analyzing, and concluding.

When information and knowledge are synthesized with feelings in direct experience, we may arrive at wisdom—the mind of the soul, a flowing and spontaneous feeling intelligence. This wisdom is effortless and able to tap into whatever is required in any moment. It is directly connected to the life force, having its own innate feeling intelligence. The fourth quality of the mind, perfect knowing, is based on emptiness. It arises spontaneously when you are empty, and it can be applied in every situation and all aspects of existence. Yet one can never own it or hold on to it. Like water, it flows and penetrates; it is always shifting in every form and situation.

In this context when you experience an insight—an "aha moment" or a new realization—you have a moment of transformation and understanding. Maybe it will last a second, a minute, a month, or a lifetime. Yet for that space of time, you recognize the truth. This is a real gift, and you often cherish it in that moment. But then your ego mind gets too involved. It starts to assume that because a deeper part of you experienced the truth, *it* also knows the truth. Then the truth of your immediate experience gets pushed back into your mind as an idea, as a memory, as a new rule to live by.

The mind may further reduce and catalog the truth down to a bit of data, an intellectual piece of information. The truth and love inherent within your realization get lost, as your mind tells you that *it* knows the truth, cleverly blocking you from following the deeper feeling of the soul and its innate knowing. In following this deeper feeling, you actually *live* the truth as it arises in any given moment because you are present with what you are really feeling.

Remember the ego mind's assumption that it knows the truth is separate from an actual experience of truth that arises during your moments of complete presence and soulful feeling. *Walking the walk is different from talking the talk.* Through your actions and experience you arrive at wisdom, a rhythmic intelligence found in the present moment, which is fluid, spontaneous, and not bound to any rules.

The mind as a servant of the soul is in its rightful place and then it is a good tool. Always keep it in third place, behind God and your own soul. This is intelligence. The mind becomes a tool for the soul to express, organize, structure, and manifest the soul's vision, the soul's purpose, the soul's passion here on Earth. The mind as servant of the soul means it is there to do the bidding of the soul.

When this is integrated, you won't have to think about things most of the time—you will just do them gracefully and automatically. You will be able to answer e-mails, pay bills, and do mental tasks without thinking or getting caught in judgments or analysis. You will act precisely, efficiently, and quickly, because the mind is the servant. When you use the mind to structure or plan things, you will think with your heart. You will think about how to be compassionate, how to put the heart into a plan of action, and how to apply love in your life.

Intelligence is part of the mind of light. This mind is about the infrastructure that keeps everything in order and harmony with perfect rhythm. Without structure, there would be no rhythmic intelligence, just a haphazard collection of cacophonic notes that sound really bad. So with the intelligent use of the mind's infrastructure, you create boundaries, which are necessary to allow form to manifest and for intelligence to flow. This allows you to be whole and to manifest who you are. It also supports your emotional core and center.

Through its light organizing principles, intelligence grounds higher visions and concepts into a usable form that we can utilize here and now. Intelligence is focused in a relaxed, aware way, not in an intense, rigid *mental* way. Your intelligent focus is one-pointed, and with true one-pointedness comes deep relaxation as well. If you meditate and pray and are accustomed to entering altered states, it can be easy for you to go into a relaxed and focused state of mind.

Intelligence needs direction, focus, function, and purpose to be able to express properly. Without this, it will become a fluffy mess or a chaotic maelstrom of thoughts and emotions. Intelligence eloquently articulates all aspects and facets of a problem, a situation, a subject, or theme, just as an expert teacher can take one word and explain succinctly what could take twenty pages of writing. When the facets of your mind are clear, then the intelligent geometry of light shines through them.

Intelligence can penetrate any body of knowledge. It can follow the threads and see the depth and truth of any subject without knowing it beforehand or being trained in it. In the brilliance of natural intelligence, you can know what you need to know at any moment. Rhythmic intelligence crafts a perfect order, where everything is in its right place and everyone is doing the right thing in harmony with everyone else.

Holy Prayer

✦

Beloved Father Mother God, please help me clear and open my mind so it becomes a transparent vessel for my soul. Help me make my mind a servant of my soul! Help me remember to follow my soul's intelligence in all the actions I do. Amen.

§ Sacred Action

Beloved One, are too many thoughts filling your head? Are you confused, divided, and doubtful? Are you masking any unfelt emotions?

Take a moment now to befriend your soul. When you find yourself thinking too much—stop, take a pause, breathe, and ask yourself: what emotions am I not feeling now? Then sink into the emotion with your breath and presence.

When the emotion is felt and released, your mind will become clear and still, allowing your soul's intelligence to shine through and be heard.

Then take action on what you've heard!

KING*

> **King**—the male ruler of a sovereign self or state; one who owns and lives his sovereignty and power in union with the feminine and to help others

As this process of divinization takes root within you, feelings of disempowerment, impotence, doing things against your will, and being unable to speak or act the truth become impossible to endure. This is

---

*This pearl, which is mainly directed toward men, is parallel to the Queen pearl (page 50), which is mainly directed toward women. Of course everyone can gain from reading and absorbing the importance of both pearls for the masculine and feminine essences inside all of us.

one sign the King is birthing within you. For this quality to anchor deeply, claim and husband this virtue by taking on the characteristics of a King and applying them every day.

In Kings there is something about their aura, their charisma, how they hold themselves, and how they speak, that makes it natural for other people to respect, admire, and want to follow them. Now *all* men being birthed into the new paradigm are being prompted by the evolutionary force within their own soul to develop and embody kingly qualities.

One of the first steps to becoming a King is to understand how to harness your gifts and attributes and use them in the right way. While there is no set list of things that make a man a King, there are certain traits that a lasting King *does* have.

The first trait that makes a good King is that he leads, and he leads by example. The second trait is that a King accepts responsibility for the positive acts *and* the errors he makes, dealing with the consequences humbly and effectively. The third trait is that when a decision needs to be made, he will make it, even if the decision is a difficult one. He stands by his decisions with a powerfully unshakable presence that others respect. Many other traits of the King, such as honor and being a pillar, are found throughout this book.

The King clearly understands his role: for his own soul to rule over his mind and wounded self, first and foremost. This he then applies to his kingdom, his world and web of relationships, soul purpose, the physical world, and other beings. The King is only crowned when all parts of himself are united in a noble calling to something far beyond himself. In this quest a man encounters all that a King is and is not.

In ancient Egypt Osiris, or Asar, was the archetypal King. His fourteen aspects correspond to the fourteen parts of his body that were cut up and deposited in various locations around Egypt before he was resurrected through the love and magic of Ast, or Isis.

The following are some of the main aspects of the King and the Divine Masculine as derived from Asar.

♦ The ability to sustain the body-mind and soul by knowing one's self; the processes and needs that are necessary to sustain endurance, stamina, and the ability to see something through until its end, which take nurturing, attention, and discipline

- The ability to nurture the body-mind and soul through right relationships, healthy internal and external environments, true speech, right conduct, and integrity
- The creative power of food and greenness—an energetic quality in you that is a living link to the spirit of the Earth and its voice, living with Nature, recycling, being zero-waste, eating organic living foods and herbs that activate and nurture the body and provide pleasure, and relating to the web of life and interconnection
- The ability to penetrate a situation, person, or thought process with clarity and insight, to reveal the inherent truth in it and to cut through any veils of illusion; this could also be called deconstructing thought processes and ideas with a penetrating or diamond mind that then serves growth through the shedding of old beliefs and ways of being
- The ability to cut through illusion with power and sever connections or create connections
- The capacity to sit in a holy state of consciousness, to command respect through your presence and accomplishments—this may not be just in the spiritual arena, as many people who have achieved a lot through age or material accomplishments also have a certain aura and resilience the vital spark of their physical being, or what the ancient Egyptians would call their Ka body
- The ability to use power to get something done when the time is right; the ability to be a leader and take charge; the ability to break down and break through any and all obstacles
- The ability to consider all aspects of a situation and others and their feelings—seeing other points of view—and then to act decisively and accordingly
- The power to be honorable, patient, and kind; to tell the truth and be honest and humble as a form of empowerment; the power to stick with honesty, honor, and integrity when everyone else is not; the ability to be strong in this no matter what temptations

are presented and the ability to live in truthful integrity, what the ancient Egyptians would call Ma'at

- The power to know your own worth and the worth of others—self-worth means loving, nurturing, and valuing one's self and being centered in sovereign self-authority, -knowing, and -leadership
- The power of radiance—the ability to radiate light and knowing to others through the combination of power and heart
- The power of illumination—the ability to illuminate any shadow, any darkness, any confusion in self or others; to light up, move, inspire, and catalyze others and yourself into action, clarity, and well-being
- The power of splendor, to be the royal being that you are, to sit in your presence, which is naturally royal and the ruler of the lower aspects of your self; to be majestic and not be ashamed of it; to be splendid without egoic attachment or concern; to sit naturally in your kingly self, the royal self that serves others; to be the center of your kingdom, for true self to be the center of your universe around which everything else revolves
- The power to wield magic; the ability to change, alchemize, and manifest situations, people, and abilities; the ability to make the impossible possible

Holy Prayer

✝

Beloved Father Mother God, You created me to be a King, one who desires to embody the Divine Masculine qualities listed above. I am ready to accept my responsibilities and claim the gifts You have placed within my soul. I am willing to lead my life through my sovereign soul and to make decisions that reflect and uphold nobility. I am burning and steadfast in my desire. Thank You, Beloved God, for helping me know and feel truth, power, and virtue. I and my Father are one. I and my Mother are one. Together we make anew all Creation. Amen.

✸ Sacred Action

Beloved One, take some time now to breathe and embody the King that you are rightfully becoming. Here is a breathing practice that allows you to feel all the aspects of your masculine essence, as you become a pillar of light and breath united and whole within yourself. The more you are centered in this, the more you will feel your self. This is especially beneficial to practice before making love, as all parts of you will become engaged, present, virile, and open.

Breathe seven times into the tip and the lips of your lingam—the tip of your sacred sword. As you feel tingling here, continue.

With your breath, connect this energy into the seed of both of your testes, your biological light generators, until they start to tingle. Breathe this loop seven times.

With your breath, connect this energy into your prostate gland seven times, deep in your body, until you feel a deep and rooted centering in this, your male power.

With your breath, connect this energy into your hara, place of power and aloneness, seven times.

With your breath, connect this energy into both of your nipples, your magnetic antennae, seven times.

With your breath, connect this energy into your chin chakra, seat of your royal authority, seven times.

With your breath, connect this energy into your alta major—the energy center at the base of your skull—entry point of Shakti, seven times.

With your breath, connect this energy into your pineal chakra, your illuminated command and vision center, seven times.

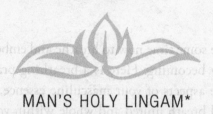

MAN'S HOLY LINGAM*

Lingam—the phallus, a symbol of divine generative energy and the beginning and end of the tantric King

The healed and consecrated lingam is a tool for love, a literal wand of light when it is fully connected to the heart of the man whose heart is connected to the soul of God. The wand of light describes the field of activated light around the lingam that is love based. It is this field that enters the womb and ignites it. Touching and kissing such a lingam brings a woman to an honoring, cherishing adoration of her partner, and love flows through her spontaneously to the man and his lingam. She, in turn, feels honored and full of gratitude for this flow of spontaneous love and connection from him.

The healed and sacred lingam is open, supple, flexible, not disposed to lust or violent entry or usage; it is a servant of love. It is not rigid, overly hard, and stiff. It can bend and fit into any opening, filling it completely with its body of light, no matter its physical size. This field fills up a woman's entire body. This wand of light penetrates into the womb itself, becoming a pillar, filling the woman completely from yoni through to crown and beyond. Ejaculation becomes a sacred act where the woman feels her partner's pure essence and exults in it, wants it, and tastes his juices through her yoni into her mouth. By its simple beingness, the holy lingam invites the woman to adore, cherish, and love it.

In making love with a healed lingam much more healing and deep connection happens. The union of lingam and yoni-womb means that neither is felt as separate: they both fit perfectly into each other and lose

---

*This pearl, which is mainly directed toward men, is parallel to the Woman's Holy Yoni pearl (page 84), which is mainly directed toward women. Of course everyone can gain from reading and absorbing the importance of both pearls for the masculine and feminine essences inside all of us.

their individual selves in this harmony. As this is happening, the yoni and womb open more, and the woman wishes to create more space within her to give all of herself to this man and to something far bigger than this man: to God. When she is filled by the light of a healed lingam, a woman can totally surrender and receive her partner's masculinity into the deepest place of her being, married with her passionate desire for the Divine, this penetrates and fulfills her completely. Seeing, feeling, and experiencing a healed lingam opens the heart of a woman to a place of trust and reverence. All her past fears or issues with men can dissolve as she returns to her original innocence and playfulness, reawakening her longing to give herself completely in open vulnerability and surrender. Making love with a man who is comfortable and assured in his heart's power, masculine essence, emotions, and sexuality allows a woman to safely feel her deepest emotions around her own sexual and emotional nature in ways that therapy or nonsexual healing can never reach.

The power wielded by a man with a healed and holy lingam is immense. He uses it to open and serve his partner and to bring great joy and bliss to his partner as well as himself. He is still and clear as he feels deeply into his partner's yoni and womb and opens up every part of her with his lingam power and heartfelt energy. Women adore this and will always want more. When a woman feels this, her whole body, emotions, and soul scream a resounding "Yes!"

He holds the space of the pillar inside her to allow her to exult, open, release, and become who she is. Through this his soul is more deeply embedded into his body. All of this is possible through the man being centered in his soul and using his I Am or his true presence to guide the lovemaking.

Holy Prayer

————————✦————————

Beloved Father Mother God, I am ready to heal my lingam of all negative emotions recorded in it. Infuse my lingam with Your divine generating energy, so I may be able to bring my heart's presence into the act of love. Help me feel and release my lust, my anger, my need for control, my selfishness, so I may become a real man. I desire to be a King of the new paradigm, shepherding in the new age of divinity within myself and all beings. Amen.

❧ Sacred Action

Look at your lingam when it is aroused.

Now visualize a sheath of light around it. Feel it. This is the light body of your lingam, and it is this part of you that enters your partner's womb and brings her to the depths of bliss and fulfillment.

Breathe into this light sheath twelve times. What do you feel?

Now, breathe this light into your heart and connect the heart and the lingam. What do you feel now?

ORCHESTRATOR

Orchestrator—one who plans or coordinates elements, forces, circumstances, or people to produce a desired effect

Orchestrators see all the pieces of a puzzle and bring them all together in harmony to achieve a symphony. They are like choir directors: they choose the pieces to be sung, assign groups of people to each specific melody and lyric, and combine them all into a harmony that brings forth perfection and beauty.

Orchestrators have similar qualities to generators, because not only do they direct, but they also assign and arrange. They may even start a creative project or relationship. They find the right people to do the right job and oversee the whole process. They assign different parts of themselves to do the right tasks, and their consciousness oversees them all, keeping them in check and balancing them so every part is working to fulfill its specific purpose. Orchestrators lovingly oversee the interactions and interconnections so vital for creating a successful company, creative project, or personal relationship. With this orchestration, all is in balance, so work and life proceed in harmony and success.

In Sacred Relationship the orchestrator is responsible for creating an ever-expanding field of awareness *in front of* his or her partner to pave the way for the divine couple, allowing them to step into this field and keep on growing—spiritually, soulfully, and emotionally. Organizing and planning for contingencies and eventualities, the orchestrator's foresight sees things before they happen, before taking action. The orchestrator is an opener of the way, a navigator.

Orchestrators smooth things over, creating more spaciousness physically, emotionally, and soulfully. Through this creating of space more can happen, more possibilities can manifest. Spaciousness is vital for any relationship as it allows both people to feel free and express themselves without worrying what the other may think or do. Emotional spaciousness allows emotions to unfold and be felt. Mental spaciousness allows new concepts, ideas, and creations to be revealed. Soulful spaciousness allows more honor, gratitude, and love to bloom as well as deeper parts of the soul to come alive. Spaciousness allows one to breathe and bloom.

Orchestrators have to be determined and focused, yet allow all parts of the whole to feel autonomous and free to enjoy their part fully. Spaciousness allows each note, each emotion, each task, and each person to rest in the space after the note is sounded, therefore finding his or her full resonance and completeness.

There are many aspects to Sacred Relationship, both within one's own self and the living field of the container between both people that bonds both souls together. Orchestrators see where they need to grow in each part of themselves: body, sexuality, emotions, mind, relating capacities, God connection, life force flow, and shadow. They tune themselves to get the best from each part, so each part is singing well, and singing together from the same sheet music, with the same goal and purpose. Then, as a tuned instrument, they can help orchestrate their relationships; they can orchestrate others in projects and creative ventures.

Each person is a symphony, a collection of individual notes playing together in a self-contained harmony. Some people know their own theme and can play it clearly and dynamically. Those with deep souls have many notes to play with; they are easy to get along with as they share a resonant sympathetic chord with our own music. Other people are complex and difficult to understand immediately because they have different chord structures from our own. These are people you might have to spend some time with before you can catch on to their music.

We feel another's music instantly—we know whether the person feels resonant to us and whether he or she fits naturally in our own symphony. We can also recognize when he or she is being true to his or her own vibration and is playing it without disguise or added notes, without pretence or falseness.

Since we are music, we have to work out how to play our theme. Ask yourself: What is my key note; what is my resonant chord? What tempos, what rhythms do I move to? What is the song of my soul? Perhaps some people have more complicated melodies, and it might be harder for them to find their groove and play them. Maybe some people find it easier to play what other people want to hear from them, as they have not yet discovered their own music.

When we get stuck in life, caught in a negative emotional pattern, it is because one or more of our notes is not being heard; it is frozen within us—a music that is not alive or expressed. Here, in this stuck place, we are not tuning in to our resonance, our truth.

In the true symphony of the Ultimate Orchestrator, God, separation between subject and object dissolves. You are not separate from him, the tree, or the person that stands before you. Your music is in harmony. Life and synchronicity are part of the field of divine orchestration, which is bringing you everything you need to be whole and helping you to experience that wholeness in your relationship.

Holy Prayer

✦

Beloved Father Mother God, help me bring together all parts of myself. Help me weave and orchestrate all my aspects of being together through the one rhythm of my soul. Show me what I need to do to unlock my frozen parts. Reveal within me my chaos and unfinished business. Show me where I need to tie up loose ends. Help me to become clear and expanded—so I may access the orchestrator within me, so

I may organize, structure, and fine-tune my being, my relationship, and my holy purpose. Amen.

♪ Sacred Action

Give some more space to yourself and your partner.

Now what is your own music, your favorite tempo, your own inner rhythm that makes you feel good?

Why are you not following this every day? What is distracting you?

What do you feel is the tempo and pace of your partner? Are your tempos compatible? If not—why not? And given some time and cooperation—could they find a harmonious rhythm?

Be honest, Beloved One, and trust your inner guidance.

PILLAR*

Pillar—a person who is regarded as reliably providing essential support for something or someone

Every man has within him the sacred quality of the pillar—the anchor and rock upon which lives can be built. This is part of the male genetic makeup. Living this genetic imperative allows a man to unfold into his divine design, propelling him into the growth he always wanted, but never could put his finger on.

The true masculine is a pillar for others to lean on and confide in, a source of strength and depth that is ever present, ever reliable. He is there no matter what, living in integrity, and he would do anything for his loved ones. He is the pillar of strength his partner can rely on

---

*This pearl, which is mainly directed toward men, is parallel to the Virgin pearl (page 74), which is mainly directed toward women. Of course everyone can gain from reading and absorbing the importance of both pearls for the masculine and feminine essences inside all of us.

and always come back to. Confiding in this pillar is much more powerful for a woman than confiding to her friends and not sharing with him. Why? Because through a couple's vulnerability with each other and their true commitment, a deeper bond is created that allows both to embody true femininity and true masculinity.

A great example of how a man can be a pillar is shown in the most intense part of labor, when just before pushing the baby out, a woman will sometimes say, "I can't!" or "It's too much!" This is when her partner moves in close, holds her hands, looks in her eyes, and lends her his strength. This allows the expectant mother to share in his strength, his solidity, his unmoving pillar, and to reaccess her own strength. He is a pillar, a solid rock, which encourages her to travel deeper into herself and release her untapped power.

The male pillar anchors and firmly grounds a relationship so that he and his partner can open to the primal powers of sex, soul, and God that are unleashed in full-blooded, lovingly committed relating. This grounded field is vital in order to maintain the integrity and safety of what is being healed and created.

The pillar keeps everything in its right place, both physically and in the realms of consciousness. He keeps things stable, linking heaven to Earth, securing and connecting one to the other. One meaning of *husband* is to wisely manage. A husband or pillar wisely manages his household, cultivating the relating, bringing life into the field of the relationship, keeping it fresh so new life and new opportunities can happen.

The pillar—solid, steady, and true—brings simplicity to the dance of relating, continually bringing himself and his partner back to their own respective center points. He puts everything into perspective, helping each individual understand the larger context. He helps his partner (or his own inner feminine) return to her soul's truth, passion, and purpose when she is caught up in the emotional swirls of her own process. He brings her back to the solid container of trust. He sees and holds the big picture, allowing both souls to find their own flows and unique expressions. He is the reminder, the balance point in the middle of it all.

The pillar is solidified through true commitment. Only then can a man step into this sacred role. The pillar speaks truth to his partner at the right times. He guides and grounds the overall energy of the relationship. He is the one whom his partner and inner feminine can rely on both internally and externally when the inner or outer world changes and parts of it come crashing down.

However, there is a balance here. Too much focus on the responsibility to be a strong pillar for everyone can stop a man from being vulnerable and human. He can become frozen, no longer flowing with his emotions, becoming isolated and trapped in a role. If a man cries and expresses his vulnerability, he may fear his partner will feel unsteady and scared around him and perceive that he is no longer the rock she can lean on. He may feel he has neglected his duty and responsibility by dropping his façade of invulnerability.

Yet a man with a façade cannot be a true pillar. A man must remember that in taking *false* responsibility for others, he can deny others their important lessons for growth and empowerment. When a man ceases to flow with and embrace the movements of his own emotions in order to be a static pillar that everyone and everything depends on, he loses a part of himself. Therefore, to be truly strong and whole, a man can allow himself to cry. He can be gentle with himself and share openly with others. When a man can communicate and create space to be alone, it allows him to drop deep into the vulnerable heart, which becomes the true foundation for the pillar to rest on. The true pillar protects and preserves the sanctity of his own inner environment as well as the environment of his home. With caring power, he stands strong in his intention to keep his partner safe from his own and others' negative thoughts, emotions, and physical aggression.

Whatever it takes to protect the environment of relationship with your partner and the Divine—do it! Your courage and power to speak out and stand up to authority is important, so your partner feels safe and can trust you are strong enough to protect her and keep her from harm. When she can let go physically and emotionally, with spirit and soul, she will respect you immensely and trust you even more. Trust is the foundation of intimacy, and love is the greatest protection. It keeps all harm at bay. From this perspective, any harm that does arise is from a lack of love in both or one of the partners.

It is important to remember that your partner's womb and yoni are sacred. Take special care of this sacred space and portal. Protect your partner's integrity (and your intimate relationship). Do not give your power and knowing away to anyone else.

The masculine, in its pure, whole, healed presence, is a pillar that needs nothing, not even relationship, while the feminine is more about relationship and interconnection. Yet life is a dance of masculine and feminine; both can happen at the same time. A man needs to integrate and experience his full femininity before he can become the true masculine, and a woman needs to integrate and experience her full masculinity in order to become the true feminine. There is a balance to be had between both aspects of the protector in the journey to become the Divine Human.

Holy Prayer

✦

Beloved Father Mother God, please help me become a pillar of strength and solidity for myself and for my partner/feminine self. Help me feel and release my fear, my impulse to run away, my fight, my weakness, and all my emotions of feeling unsupported and alone. Help me feel and release all my abandonment wounds with my own mother and father. Help me to release the burdens carried within my masculine self including having to go out there into the world to make my mark as a man to other men. Help me to lay down my burdens, to become cleansed and purified by the feminine (my feminine) essence. Help me to release my aggression, force, and sheer will so I may be in the world, but not of it. For I, the Divine Masculine—am here! Amen.

♪ Sacred Action

Beloved One, lay down your burdens and come together with the feminine (your feminine partner or feminine self) and let go. It is time for you to receive some cleansing from the gentleness of the Mother and far-reaching love from your lover.

Turn to the alchemical body practice "The Sacred Prostitute" and embody her wisdom and his rebirth.

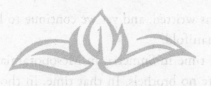

ALCHEMICAL BODY PRACTICE

THE SACRED PROSTITUTE

I was sent forth from the power,
and I have come to those who reflect upon me,
and I have been found among those who seek after me,
Look upon me, you who reflect upon me,
and you hearers, hear me.
You who are waiting for me, take me to yourselves
And do not banish me from your sight . . .
For I am the first and the last
I am the honored one and the scorned one,
I am the whore and the holy one . . .
I am the silence that is incomprehensible
and the idea whose remembrance is frequent.
I am the voice whose sound is manifold
and the word whose appearance is multiple.
I am the utterance of my name . . .

FROM "THE THUNDER, PERFECT MIND,"
THE NAG HAMMADI LIBRARY

So opens "The Thunder, Perfect Mind." This short tractate is part of the Nag Hammadi library. It is the proclamation of the great female I-Am. Throughout the piece this powerful voice utters apparent paradoxes that stretch opposites into truth.

"The Thunder, Perfect Mind" speaks in the voice of a divine female power. She asserts her importance to a people who were already deeply ambivalent about her: a people whose ancestors had been torn for centuries between honoring and scorning her. This female I-Am knows that the people are on the verge of forgetting who she is and becoming deaf to her wisdom. Some 1,800 years have passed since "The Thunder,

Perfect Mind" was written, and yet we continue to hear her, this voice whose sound is manifold.

Once upon a time in Sumeria, in Mesopotamia, in Egypt, and in Greece, there were no brothels. In that time, in those countries, there were temples of the sacred prostitutes. In these temples men were cleansed, not sullied, morality was restored, not desecrated, and sexuality was not perverted, but divine.

The original whore was a priestess, a conduit of the divine. One could enter the Sacred through her body and be restored. Warriors and others soiled by combat within the world of men came to the holy prostitute, the Quedishtu, literally meaning "the undefiled one." By sharing the sexual act with her in a sacred temple, they were cleansed and reunited with Source through pleasure and prayer—essential attributes that pleased the gods. Originally these holy prostitutes were revered as a doorway to God. They were not victims, nor were they forced into prostitution as many women and young girls are today. They willingly took on the office of priestess and acted from an empowered place of divine service.

The first patriarchs, the priests of Judea and Israel and the prophets of Jehovah, condemned the holy prostitutes and their worship of Asherah, Astarte, Anta, and other ecstatic goddesses. Morality was the pretext behind which the patriarchs consolidated ecclesiastic power. Fear of the wild, ecstatic energy of the Feminine was perhaps a hidden reason; the Goddess in her power was difficult to control. And so, as patriarchy came to rule the world, priests systematically replaced women priestesses as intermediaries between men and God.

What was the impact of the suppression of the holy prostitute?

Hades, the spiritual center of Greek paganism, became hell. The descent into Hades, which was at the core of the Eleusinian Mysteries and a spiritually required initiation for anyone concerned with soul, was prohibited. By the middle of the fourth century, the Christians had suppressed these mysteries and installed hell as a place of punishment and torture. People could be saved from hell only by following the dictates of Christian priests.

Furthermore the sacred union teachings of Jesus and his wife Mary

Magdalene, herself a former temple priestess, were twisted and all but lost. Only chastity and celibacy were considered pure and holy. The body was considered impure, and some people whipped themselves or wore hair shirts to mortify the flesh. Procreation was infused with anxiety and guilt, while joyful fertility festivals, which had provided a link between Earth and Spirit, were condemned as shameful orgies. Men returned from war without the ability to clean the blood from their hands, engendering post-traumatic stress disorders that have grown over the centuries like a malignant cancer.

When the priests separated the body and its delight from the gods, they separated God from Nature, and thereby created the mind-body split. With this paradigm shift, the world became secularized. The consequences have rippled through humanity ever since. Not only were the sacred prostitutes exiled, but also the gods. Perhaps the world as we have come to know it—impersonal, abstract, detached, brutish—was born in that division. In a sacred universe the Earth is a loving mother who must be treated with respect; the prostitute is a holy woman—one whose love, kindness, and sensuality restores, redeems, and rebirths. When the Goddess of Love, the female I-Am was still honored, the sacred prostitute was virgin in the original sense of the word: whole within herself. She was a person of deep strength and integrity, whose welcome for the stranger was radiant, self-confident, and sensuous. Her purpose was to bring the Goddess's love into direct contact with mankind. In antiquity human sexuality and a religious attitude were inseparable.

In our fragmented times our vitality and capacity for joy depend on restoring the soul of the sacred prostitute to its rightful place in our conscious understanding. She reminds us how human sexuality and its relationship to the well-balanced personality restores—almost overnight—the health and stability of human society. She embodies the wholeness that is so needed now.

The sacred prostitute is still with us, and her consorts still feel the longing for her initiation. Those of us who know and honor her must reinstate her divine act of love, not only to its original glory, but to a brilliant new height appropriate for the new paradigm we are co-creating. But first we must heal the wounds of the old paradigm.

Healing the Sacred Prostitute
and Her Consort

Many of us *know* we carry the energy of the sacred prostitute. We carry the rites of the temple in our soul consciousness and feel intuitively that we are here on Earth to embody this work again. There are also those of us who *know* we are here to be initiated by a sexual experience that reveals the essence of God within our own soul.

I (Padma) have traveled the world and met so many people who feel this way. In our conversations I discovered the same thing invariably happened for all of these people: first, people experienced unbridled grief, then a powerful release of guilt, shame, and loneliness, followed by waves of overwhelming love that poured out through tender words and acts of compassion, kindness, and profound peace. I have witnessed this again and again.

Eventually, I realized that the Universe was asking me to open a space for the sacred prostitute to be redeemed and baptized by her consort, and for her consort to be anointed by her bodhisattva compassion and virgin love.

Here is a practice that you can do with a partner or by yourself. I advise doing both, so you may have the experience of receiving love from another human being and also from the divine source deep within your being.

❧ Step One

Put on some tender and heartfelt background music.

Come into a comfortable cross-legged position, either facing your partner or sitting by yourself.

Lift your heart in prayer, asking to connect with the energies of either the sacred prostitute or consort inside of you.

If you are connecting to the sacred prostitute, now is the time to bravely reach in and retrieve her. She has had to hide for so long, and she may feel terribly alone, exiled, forbidden, suppressed, excommunicated, and fearful. She may also have feelings of outrage, anger, fury, revenge, or deep, deep sadness, acute pain, and sorrow. Whatever arises, welcome it with an open and kind heart.

If you are connecting to the consort, you may experience feelings of guilt, shame, distrust, suspicion, or grief. Again, go with it and keep your heart open.

Use your breath and prayer to authentically connect to these parts within.

If you are doing this work alone, you are being asked to work with your inner sacred prostitute and consort—aspects of your inner feminine and masculine energies. As you continue to read, hold this concept inside and follow the same guidance as if your sacred other was present. The only difference is that you will be doing everything on the inside.

Before we can move to the next stage, the consort has to indicate when the time is right. The consort needs to feel strong, centered, and anchored during this retrieval process. With an open heart, the consort is invited to love and behold the sacred prostitute in the past, present, and future—throughout all time and space. This means breathing through all judgment, shame, and fear until all that is left is an expanding pillar of luminous love force.

◗ Step Two

The consort now comes forward and holds the sacred prostitute in a position where she can really let go. This may be spooning one another on the floor, or the consort may be holding the sacred prostitute's belly from behind as the consort's back is supported against a wall. It doesn't matter how it looks; what matters is how it feels.

The sacred prostitute needs to feel held, supported, loved, and protected—so she may release all the wounds associated with this archetype and the fear of embodying her gifts.

The sacred prostitute is invited to take long, slow breaths to reach the dark bottom of this ancient archetype, sinking down into her body-mind system to feel what is there. With the luminous presence and support of the consort, she now bestows love and healing to this exiled sense of self.

Before we can move to the next stage, the sacred prostitute has to indicate when the time is right. She also needs to feel strong, centered, and anchored in this retrieval process. Grounded in her own worthiness, and with an open heart, the sacred prostitute is invited to behold the consort in the past, present, and future—throughout all time and space. This means breathing through all judgment, shame, and fear until all that is left is a tender, compassionate heart radiant with luminous love force.

❧ Step Three

The sacred prostitute now comes forward and holds her consort in a position where he can really receive. She may sit on top of him as he is lying down (see below) or with both partners seated in the yab-yum position (see next page).

The sacred prostitute can stroke the consort's skin, gently massaging and caressing the tension out of his being. Because of the earlier healing, she is now fully able to embody the sacred prostitute and be brave and tender at the same time. She can fully let go and allow her instinctual loving essence to move through her.

The consort is invited to receive her healing caresses deep down into his cells, into his brain, and into his DNA, erasing every memory from the past and any projections of fear of the future. He remains in the present now.

Every breath the sacred prostitute and consort take together is anointed with the healing grace of love, light, and comfort.

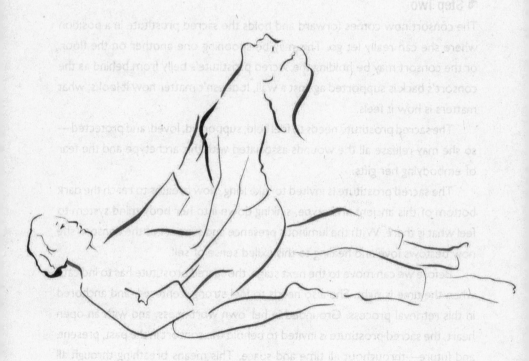

**The lying down position for the
sacred prostitute practice**

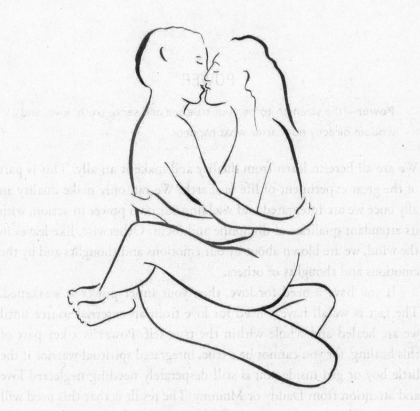

The yab-yum position for the
sacred prostitute practice

If you are doing this practice alone, touch, soothe, caress, and hold yourself so you can send healing waves of compassion to the inner masculine consort.

As the qualities of the sacred prostitute continue to guide and inspire you, remember how she used all of her body to love, bless, comfort, and nurture the consort. Her hands, her eyes, her breath, her voice, her yoni, her womb, her tears, her mind, and her heart all worked together in this sacred dance.

Love with the whole of your body. May the grace of Her be with you always.

Amen.

POWER

Power—the strength to be your true self and serve truth, love, and wisdom directly no matter what happens

We are all here to learn from duality and make it an ally. This is part of the great experiment of life on Earth. We can only make duality an ally once we are integrated and wielding our own power in action, with its attendant qualities of discipline and focus. Otherwise, like leaves in the wind, we are blown about by our emotions and thoughts and by the emotions and thoughts of others.

If you have a need for love, then your inner power is weakened. The fact is we all have a need for love from an external source until we are healed and whole within the true self. Power is a key part of this healing, for you cannot be a true, integrated spiritual warrior if the little boy or girl inside you is still desperately needing neglected love and attention from Daddy or Mommy. The result is that this need will be projected onto your partner. This early wounding must be lovingly tended to and healed before true power can bloom.

When you are centered in inner power in the core of your hara or womb, you can clearly discern things and have healthy emotional boundaries, for you know yourself. You have spent time by yourself cultivating your power, getting to know it. You have tried it out in real life situations as well as by yourself with your own discipline and your own mindfulness.

When you are firmly rooted in your own personal power, no one can bring you off balance. To inquire and think for your self takes inner power—it takes strength, energy, and a certain penetrative quality. Without inner power you end up ungrounded, a sheep following the crowd rather than following your own soul. Your mind is full of other people's beliefs, collective beliefs, New Age beliefs, and so on. You will project on others your disowned qualities of power and strength, and you will not like other people who have these qualities, because you disown them within yourself.

Power is the quality most do not want to fully and unreservedly own. It involves taking a long hard look at yourself and your beliefs. You must examine your relationships, your ideas around what love is and what love is not, as well as your inherited beliefs around power. Many beings utilize power in order to control and manipulate large groups of human beings. Many people are scared of power because they see how power is being used on a subconscious level to harm and control. Those who manipulate power in the world create fear in order to stop people from stepping into their own power and thinking for themselves.

People who are clear in their inner power can walk away from anything or anyone, without any hesitation. In power you start to access the beginning of a consciousness that has no need. It is self-contained. This is one of the pillars, along with love and wisdom, that forms the basis for the integration of higher consciousness. If there is no need in you, then you can flow with everything.

Many Indian and Tibetan yogis use willpower, pure focus, and consistent discipline to meditate for long periods of time to open up the third eye. In India they call it the power of *tapas*—the inner fire of austerity—and *sadhana*—a spiritual practice, which opens up inner faculties such as clairvoyance, ESP, and charisma.

When you are centered in your power, you can discern. You can penetrate illusion and more than that—you possess the power to change it. You see the illusion and stop it in that moment. There are no ifs and buts, no excessive thinking. You are the sovereign ruler of your kingdom. You don't need to discuss your decisions and you don't need approval from anyone. Your sovereign self moves forward directly and dynamically because it has penetrated the illusion of your self or another. Power either ends something or begins something. Power is a dynamic movement. You are going somewhere and nothing is going to stop you. This takes discipline as well. This does not happen in just one day or one hour. The human consciousness takes time to adapt to this way of being.

Those who have integrated power are catalysts for themselves and others. They create change not to fit in to the system, but to break the system. Power can destroy. It can destroy your old life and its illusions, the falseness and insanity of yourself and the world. With this also comes the power of *no. No,* I am not going to take this anymore; *no,* I am not going to live in this illusion anymore; *no,* I am not going to put up with your bullshit anymore. *No.* Only a master can say no to anything and everything.

The greatest betrayal is to betray your soul. Do not betray your own soul. Have the power and sovereignty to stand up for yourself, to embrace your inner power, and to go for it, no matter what. Once power is integrated in you, you can effortlessly wield it in a calm, dispassionate way. You see what needs to be done and you do it. There does not need to be any emotion around it. It is a calm, clear consciousness that wields true power.

Holy Prayer

✦

Beloved Father Mother God, please help me reclaim the pieces of my personal power. Help me create change in my life with powerful purpose and direction. Help me find my inner confidence and love for myself and all the great gifts You have planted within me. Help me clean my life and all the circumstances and situations I find myself in. Thank You. Amen.

⑤ Sacred Action

Beloved One, ask yourself the following questions. To whom are you giving away your power? Are you giving power away to society, your friends, your family, your partner, the government, the law?

Why are you doing it? What are you scared of? Are you scared of the overwhelming power inside yourself? Are you afraid to unleash the mighty and awesome being that you are? Are you scared of what others will think of you if you stand up for yourself and express things they may not like? Are you scared that you will estrange yourself from your friends?

Are any of your friends in their true power? Do you know anyone in his or her true power?

Think about the above questions and then practice saying *no* in ways that empower you.

RESPONSIBILITY

Responsibility—the opportunity or ability to act independently and take decisions without the need of permission, recognition, or authorization

One of the biggest questions of life is this: will I assume responsibility for doing whatever I must do to eradicate every misperception, every obstacle to the presence of love, and every limited belief I have ever learned about anyone or anything—especially about myself?

The part of us that can accept this almighty quest is our masculine expression. It is *his* consciousness and thirst for truth that accepts this journey. The ability to be accountable, trustable, and stand for integrity are gleaming qualities that the masculine part of us loves! The masculine part of us must also be autonomous. It must be self-regulating with an eye on divine truth. We, as emerging Divine Humans, must be responsible for healing the many ways in which we may have abandoned ourselves. Responsibility can also be seen as *response-ability:* our ability to respond appropriately to any situation from our highest selves. Doing the work of healing allows us to let go of old wounded reactions and respond from a higher place. This has a positive effect on all of our relationships. When researching other pioneering voices in our community, I discovered the work of Dr. Margaret Paul and Dr. Erika Chopich, who wrote in The Inner Bonding® 7-Day Course:*

"We all have two kinds of painful feelings—our wounded feelings

---

*Reproduced from "The Free 7-Day Inner Bonding® Course" at http://www.innerbonding .com/welcome with permission from Dr. Margaret Paul and Dr. Erika Chopich. For more information on their books, workshops, and online classes visit http://www.innerbonding .com.

that we are causing with our thoughts and actions, and our existential feelings, which are the result of life. Feelings such as anger, anxiety, stress, depression, hurt, guilt, shame, frustration, emptiness, and aloneness are wounded feelings that come from our own thoughts and actions. Painful feelings such as loneliness, helplessness over others, grief, sorrow over people hurting other people, or outrage over injustice are core-self feelings. We do the Six Steps of Inner Bonding [given on page 170] when there are wounded-self feelings, and we nurture ourselves when there are core-self painful feelings.

"Our core self is our true self or essence. It is helpful to imagine the true self as a bright and shining child, the natural light within that is an individualized expression of divine love. This aspect of ourselves is actually ageless—it always has been and it always will be; it evolves through our life experiences over lifetimes. Our true self contains our unique gifts and talents, our natural wisdom and intuition, our curiosity and sense of wonder, our playfulness and spontaneity, and our ability to love and connect with others. This unwounded aspect of the soul can never be harmed. It was never touched by any abuse we suffered. Instead, this self was hidden away, covered over time by a layer of pain and false thoughts. It waits to be retrieved through a healing process. Because of this unbroken part in each of us, complete healing can occur when you have fully retrieved this aspect of yourself. Then you deeply know who you really are: a child of the unconditional love that is God. Practicing Inner Bonding leads to the reclaiming of the core Self.

"Your wounded self is the aspect that may have suffered from physical, sexual, and/or emotional abuse or neglect and it carries all the fears, false beliefs, and controlling behaviors that result from these experiences. While these fears, beliefs, and behaviors cause us pain in our adult lives, they were the only way we could feel safe when we were children. They were our survival mechanisms. Your wounded self can be any age in any given moment, depending on how old you were when you learned a particular false belief, addiction, or way to control.

"The wounded self is the aspect of you that may use food, drugs, sex, or alcohol to numb out fear and loneliness. In addition the wounded self always fears being rejected or abandoned on the one hand and being engulfed, smothered, or controlled on the other hand. In other words the wounded self fears loss of other and loss of self, because it does not know how to manage rejection without taking it personally, or to set appropriate limits against engulfment. Through anger, blame, resistance, compliance, or withdrawal, the wounded self hopes to ward off and control that which it fears. All the parts of the wounded self need healing, and they can be healed only through compassion, acceptance and unconditional love.

"The main ways we abandon ourselves in relationship are:

1. *We judge ourselves rather than accept ourselves.*
2. We ignore our feelings by staying up in our head rather than being present in our body, especially our painful feelings of loneliness, heartache, heartbreak and grief.
3. We turn to various addictions to numb the anxiety, depression, guilt, shame or anger that we cause when we judge ourselves and ignore our feelings.
4. We make others responsible for our feelings."

Our responsibility to the new paradigm calls us to the wholeness of healing the wounded self and seeking divine union.

Holy Prayer

———————✦———————

Beloved Father Mother God, help me not to blame, manipulate, or project things onto my partner. Help me remember that my partner is never responsible for my feelings. Help me to be mature and loving and take responsibility for myself and to come to You in crisis and pain. For the truth is, only You can heal me and help me uncover my true self. Help me to have the loving compassion to remind my partner gently should he or she try to place responsibility for his or her wounds on me. Help my partner and I to have integrity and honor in this process. Help us to do the work honestly and cleanly, so that we can heal our wounded inner children and all false beliefs we have around pain and suffering. Beloved God, thank You for this opportunity to become fully responsible for my own healing. Amen.

ঙ *Sacred Action*

Do you feel you have abandoned yourself? Do you blame your partner for your emotions? Do you feel anxious, fearful, tight, and disconnected?

Take the time now to look and practice the Six Steps of Inner Bonding that move us from wounding to healing. The Six Steps of Inner Bonding given below are from the 7-Day Inner Bonding Course taught by Dr. Margaret Paul and Dr. Erika Chopich.*

"Step One: *Become mindful of your feelings.* Decide that you want 100 percent responsibility for the ways in which you may be causing your own pain and for creating your own peace and joy.

"Step Two: *Choose the intent to learn to love yourself and others. Making this choice opens your heart, allows divine love in, and moves you into your loving adult self.*

"Step Three: *Choose to welcome, embrace, and dialogue with your wounded self, exploring your thoughts and false beliefs and the resulting behaviors that may be causing your pain. Bring compassion to your wounded feelings. Explore your gifts and what brings joy to your true and essential self.*

"Step Four: *Dialogue with God, discovering the truth. Think of a loving action you could make toward your self.*

"Step Five: *Take the loving action learned in step four.*

"Step Six: *Evaluate the effectiveness of your loving action. How does it make you feel? Is your true self shining more brightly?*

"These steps are actually a powerful roadmap to healing the false beliefs that may be keeping you limited in your personal life and at work."

---

*Reproduced from "The Free 7-Day Inner Bonding® Course" at http://www.innerbonding .com/welcome with permission from Dr. Margaret Paul and Dr. Erika Chopich. For more information on their books, workshops, and online classes visit http://www.innerbonding .com.

TRUTH

Truth—the quality or state of being true or real in the absolute sense

If you tell the truth, you don't have to remember anything.

MARK TWAIN

Truth goes hand in hand with love. Truth leads to more love. The more love we have realized in the substance of our soul, the more truth we live and access. The more truth we live, the more love we will have in our lives.

Truth grows in you as you speak it, express it, and share it. Truth diminishes in you when you know something and do not share it. The more you speak and share your personal truth and universal truth, the more it radiates in your life. The less you speak out and the more you hide, the more truth will shrivel in your life. Sometimes we do not want to hear the truth about ourselves or another, and we will resist it with all our might. Then the Universe/God will eventually, over time, seed the truth within us through others and certain situations, so we can surrender to that truth.

Receive truth from anyone and everyone. To resist it is your own pride and lack of desire to grow. It is not your business, or anyone else's fault, how life delivers insights that are true about you. Your learning is to receive these insights, however they are delivered, and to work through them yourself.

Receive the pain that comes with truth, no matter how unjust and unfair it may seem to be in that moment. This makes you humble. It is only painful because it lives in you already. You can justify, excuse, deny, and rationalize it, but if it is painful, it is hitting something in you that is unresolved. Accepting this pain as something within you, no matter what it appears to be *outside* of you, allows the release of it from your soul forever. This then leads to more truth.

With humility, truth will come if you deeply desire it. If you sincerely want to know the total truth about yourself, it is available to you. But you may not like it! Truth and love are two of the most maligned words in human history. Personal truths exist because of our own unique lessons on the journey from wounding into wholeness. Yet we all unite in the one truth of love.

Truth breaks us open into our naked selves. It strips away our facade and reveals our wounded self and then leads us by the hand into our shining, pure, glorious true self. Truth is aloneness: all-one-ness. The more truth we live, the less need we have for anything or anyone. The more truth we live, the more we naturally help and support others.

Truth is clarity. The more simply we can express something complex, the clearer it is. This shows we have embodied and mastered it. The more precise we are in our prayers, the more clearly we manifest them. The more succinctly we share our truth with others and describe our creative endeavors, the more successful they become and the more they are heard. Clarity sees self and others with laserlike precision. It sees the truth of who they are—beloved divine children of God—and it sees their blocks to this, the untruth of who they think they are. Clarity means being centered in your pure soul and still mind and approaching life from here. Truth is always clear.

Only a master can say *no* to anything. He or she is clear in what the universal truth is, what his or her personal truth is, and where they meet and merge. Therefore masters are empowered to say *no* because they know the truth about themselves and they understand divine truth.

The more we fearlessly investigate all parts of our self in all situations with different types of people, the more we get to know our self— and our truth. Traveling is good for this, as are Sacred Relationships, which are another form of travel.

The more we connect to Beloved God, the more we get to know divine and universal truths. Both personal truth and universal truth integrate in our journey when we are truly humble and have healed the wounds that create untruth. We approach the Divine through our own personal lens or truth, and make the Divine our own—or rather the Divine makes us in her own image when we are ready to let go of our personal truths.

Truth is individual until it becomes selfless. Truth has no self; therefore it is everywhere and nowhere. It is always flowing and available. The truth is that there is nothing to hold on to. No concept, teaching, teacher, or relationship. All of this has to go in order for you to live the truth.

Since there are no teachings, what can remain? Truth.

And you will know the truth, and the truth will set you free.

JOHN 8:32

Holy Prayer

———————————✦———————————

Beloved Father Mother God, please help me feel the naked truth about myself. I want to know where I am without truth in my life. Please help me feel all the fears I have. Please help me feel all the ways I control myself as well as others. Please help me feel the pride and unworthiness that cuts me off from Your great soul. Beloved Father Mother God, please send me Your divine truth so I may embody that. Amen.

§ *Sacred Action*

Ask yourself the following questions. Where are you out of alignment with truth right now? Where are you not following your personal truth? Where are you not following divine truth in your life?

How many times this week have you neglected to speak truth to another or yourself? How many times this week have you thought or felt a truth about yourself or another, yet failed to put it into action?

Beloved One, drop into your breathing before asking the next questions. As you reread this Pearl of Wisdom with these questions in mind, allow yourself to simply witness—and become aware of the answer that appears, much like an innocent child would simply observe, without editing, judgment, or analysis.

- What is the most significant sentence for me in this Pearl of Wisdom?
- What does that sentence mean for me?
- Is there any sentence in which I find my breath changes or that causes an emotion to arise? Causes resistance? Gets the mind racing?

- Is there any part of me that doubts, wavers, questions, or minimizes this Pearl of Wisdom?
- Am I willing to truly allow my entire existence to be full of truth?
- What shift can I make in myself that would allow this Pearl of Wisdom—and the import of its acceptance—to settle more firmly into my bones during the next two weeks? How would that shift show up in my daily life?

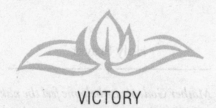

VICTORY

Victory—the act of triumphantly moving forward into a desired outcome

Having a loving relationship with a partner and God is how a human can become Divine. This act of alchemy *is* birthing the new paradigm. This arises through our own transparency, vulnerability, and passionate desire for truth, sharing our selves in a defenseless and humble way. To take this risk means we can win the victory of love.

Masks and bravado dissolve, wounds reveal, tears flow, and you are no longer pretty, perfect, strong, or powerful, or so you think. In fact you are the most beautiful and lovable at this moment, and anyone who is in his or her heart will warm to you, support you, and love you.

One needs to master the dark side, and the only way to master it is to fully experience, feel, and release it, for it is from here that a deeper compassion blooms. The victory of awakening creates beautiful people. Beautiful people are those who have suffered the most, who have known struggle, who have known loss, and who have found their way out of the depths. Beautiful people do not just happen; they are made victorious through their journey within the dark to become light.

Male-female union, inner and outer, is the basis for any true awakening and is the basis for an awakened civilization on Earth. Union between male and female is the beating heart of Christ consciousness. As Christ said in the Gospel of Thomas, "When you make the two into One, when you make the inner like the outer and the high like the low; when you make male and female into a single One, so that the male is not male and the female is not female . . . then you will enter into the Kingdom."*

You become closer with your partner by going through your own emotions alone, and at times being present with the other's shadow as a couple, *together*. This brings deeper intimacy and commitment, and it grounds love, affection, and lightness. It binds these feelings into a solid foundation of trust and presence. You know that you and your partner are there for each other through thick and thin, not just there for the good times. You accept the other, just as you accept your own flaws, without self-punishing or making the other feel bad for his or her flaws. This acceptance is part of the path to victory.

The shadow is based on grief, sadness, and pain, and it is these feelings we resist. The shadow is those darker parts of our souls that have not seen or felt the light of love. The shadow remains because neither human love, nor divine love has entered this place. The shadow is those parts of ourselves that have been unloved and unembraced—the parts of ourselves we deny and hide.

Often it is harder for us to see our own shadows, and that is where the sacred mirror of the relationship will reflect back to you all that you have denied about yourself. Just as you are committed to embracing yourself, be present with your partner in his or her anger and neediness as he or she reaches closure in accepting the shadow side; love your partner even when he or she is shut down. To remain constant in your love through these expressions of the shadow requires commitment and leads to a victorious union of deep trust and intimacy.

In simply being with the other through this—without judging, accusing, or making your *own* wounds be all about the other—more love blooms. This aids the other soul to feel deeper into his or her pain and retrieve the healing balm for it. In being present with your partner's worst pain and deepest shadow, no matter what it is, the love between you will grow exponentially and settle into a grounded, loving partnership, a victorious Sacred Relationship.

---

*From *The Gospel of Thomas: The Gnostic Wisdom of Jesus* as translated by Jean-Yves Leloup (Rochester, Vt.: Inner Traditions, 2005).

In Sacred Relationship one is naked, vulnerable, and stripped down to one's bare soul. There is a need for total transparency. It takes courage to defeat your fears. And the only way to defeat them is to express them. Sharing our deepest fears, our pain as well as our joy, is what bonds souls and leads to communion. This is the victory we are aiming for. Bravery, courage, commitment, and loyalty to truth are all aspects of this victorious spirit.

The fuel for the victorious flame of unconditional love is divine love. In order for the flames of love to burn continuously, through thick and thin, we need to have a strong link to Mother-Father God. Coupled with divine love, your human expression of love becomes alchemical: a fire of love, a burning flame fuelled and strengthened by your capacity to receive divine love and share love with your partner.

One key to supporting the flourishing of Sacred Relationship is to daily see each other as fresh and new. We can sabotage newness and the growth of the relationship by continually holding on to past hurts. By refusing to let go, we hold each other in the past and block the very change that we desire in our partner, in ourselves, and in the relationship. It is important that emotions are felt and expressed in the moment, for this avoids a stagnant build up of emotion.

When God is invited to shine light over a relationship, a sacred trinity is formed of you, your partner, and God. The relationship becomes a blessed crucible for accelerated evolution and soul growth as all three of you say *yes* to the victory of love.

Holy Prayer
✦

Beloved Father Mother God, help me to be victorious in love. Help me to align with love's voice, love's actions, and love's guidance. I am truly ready to be vulnerable, innocent, and undefended. I choose transparency. I choose healing. I choose growth. Help me to be humble to my partner's feedback and to feel into his or her observations with curiosity and willingness to not only listen, but grow. Help me Father Mother God, to share my own observations with clarity, compassion, and wisdom. Help me be able to articulate in such a way that I can be heard and be made helpful. Help me to embody the victorious virtues of courage and loyalty. Granting me the resolution to take leaps of faith when nessaccary. Thank You, God, for this ripeness within me and the grace of being willing and able to grow. Amen.

⚡ Sacred Action

Beloved One, are you feeling stuck and unable to move forward? Do you desire victory? Are you longing for a breakthrough, one that births radical transformation and liberation? This is within your grasp, my friend, and closer than you imagine. It has to be so impossibly real for our acts of faith to be exactly that. Take heart, Beloved One. Everything is happening *for* us, rather than *to* us.

Read the quote below and allow yourself to truly feel its transmission:

> *There is an almost sensual longing for communion with others who have a large vision. The immense fulfillment of the friendships between those engaged in furthering the evolution of conscious has a quality almost impossible to describe.*

> PIERRE TEILHARD DE CHARDIN

Who are the ones that trigger you to feel this way? I often feel that frustration is the other side of inspiration. Take a deep breath beloved and reach for your inspiration. You can do this! Reach out to them now and get your juices flowing. If in this moment you cannot think of others, feel into the part of yourself that you know carries a greater vision. Tune in, have courage, be loyal to its cause, and this fluidity will wash away all stagnation. Open yourself up to your creative fire and inexhaustible imagination. The victory of love is immanent.

BOOK OF ALCHEMY
Attributes of Divine Marriage

WE ARE: Pure Creation

We Are One flow of love, Embodied and Sovereign, Communicative, Listening, Committed, and Transparent, We Desire The Beloved in Holy Desire and Humility. We are The Prayer that is Rapturous.

We are a Rhythmic, Primordial Feeling of Love and Power United. Our Alchemy of Sensuality, Trust, Self-Love, and Integrity allows us both to surrender. Our Inner Children Are Friends of the Heart, and we radiate our Love and Sacred Contribution in Union.

We are The Children of Mother Father God, Creator Intelligence of Divine Love and Truth: We are the Divine Marriage.

The potency of the process known as Divine Marriage creates the birth of the Divine Human. This alchemical process ignites when the pairs of opposites, particularly masculine and feminine, fuse to create a third—the Divine Child. This child or offspring of the marriage resurrects the nobility of the Divine Masculine and radiance of the Divine Feminine in their full splendor. The balanced dance of feminine flow and masculine direction must come alive within us so we can co-create this next evolutionary stage of human existence, for this union is the foundation of an awakened civilization.

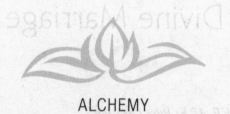

ALCHEMY

Alchemy—a magical dance of the powers of transformation that create something or someone new

True alchemy is both fiery and tender at the same time. It includes the traditional cool practices of transcendence, while blending them with the hot fires of erotic initiation and warm reverence for the Earth. The core mystery of this era is the birth of the sacred androgyne—a being filled with a hunger to fuse Heaven and Earth, masculine and feminine, stillness and action into every aspect of its existence.

The alchemy that births this Divine Human consists of four initiatory forces. These four forces are the keys that unlock the potential within life.

> **Our shamanic connection** to tribal wisdom and seasonal cycles; our compassionate connection with animals and Nature expressed as the feminine aspect of Creation
>
> **Our gnostic connection** to the transcendent peace, stillness, and freedom of the masculine aspect of Creation
>
> **Our tantric connection** to the ecstasy of the body, making love, and expressing creatively and abundantly: in essence, the mar-

riage between the masculine and feminine in ourselves and in
our relationships

Our sacred-work connection, which stirs all this into an alchemical elixir that inspires us to contribute to the Great Rebirth in a
real and tangible way

Beloved Friend, if you can weave all this together in your life, first
with yourself and then with your beloved, you shall be accessing the
pioneering force that will birth you. This alchemical elixir is really
rather simple—after all, it is composed of four joyful ingredients. The
only obstacle that could prevent us from accessing these qualities is the
lure of the old paradigm. This mind-set puts work first and compassion,
purpose, growth, and passion last. In the new paradigm work becomes
unified with our highest purpose and passion. It all flows together in a
joyous and satisfying alchemical dance. We discover our gifts and give
them to the world. This is our work, our soul's mission. In this new
paradigm life we spend time in Nature; we balance prayerful solitude
with Sacred Relationship and community celebration.

So—find out what you love to do, and with a massive leap of faith,
just do it! Add some patience and prayer, and a new alchemy will bloom
in you that will be both courageous and thrilling. Before you know it,
you will be on your way—a Divine Human with a first-class ticket to
the new paradigm!

Holy Prayer
✦

*Beloved Mother Father God, help me to love myself so tenderly
and deeply that I place my holy purpose, passion, and growth as
the number one priority in my life. Help me to embody the divine
light of life so I may live fully and completely—creating, growing,
experiencing, learning, developing, and tasting all that You have
created. Dearest God, help me become free from the controlling
methods and ways of this patriarchal era, so I may enter the love
and unity consciousness that is occurring on this glorious planet
now. Help me to have faith and to trust in You completely. You*

created me to thrive and give my gifts! Help me to integrate in sacred alchemy. Help me open my shamanic connection, my gnostic connection, my tantric connection, and my connection to sacred work. I am so grateful for this life, and I choose to deeply share my essence with all of Creation. Amen.

§ Sacred Action

Create an illustration that maps and navigates the four initiatory forces above into their own sections.

Place your different personal activities into the four quarters. For example, high vibration nutrition could go in the shamanic quarter, Vipassana meditation could go in the gnostic quarter, dance and festivals could go in the tantric quarter, and creative brainstorming about your mission could go in the sacred work quarter.

Then write answers to the following questions.

- When you think of yourself becoming a Divine Human, what are you most excited about?
- How does Sacred Relationship fit in with your vision of your highest self?
- What is your goal in life? Now double it. What is the version of the goal that is so big you are afraid to admit, even to yourself, for fear of failure?
- What's holding you back?
- What support do you need to move forward?
- What simple, concrete step would make the biggest impact to move you forward?
- Imagine you have achieved your desire. Spend a few moments really feeling that completion. How do you feel?
- Close your eyes and ask each major decision making system for advice: What does your head say? What does your heart say? What does your womb/hara say? If they are at odds, have a conversation. Can you reconcile the three?
- Dig even deeper. What do you really desire—if you could do *anything at all,* with *no* limits, what would it be?

What are you waiting for? Take one concrete action now! Take another tomorrow . . .

Let the alchemy begin!

COMMITMENT

> **Commitment**—being dedicated in integrity to a cause, activity, pledge, or person

A committed relationship is one in which two souls support each other in being whole, complete individuals. The commitment is to going all the way—letting the relationship be a catalyst for the individuals to live into and express their full potential, wisdom, love, and creativity. A committed relationship is committing to truth, love, your sovereign self, *and* your beloved other. All qualities support each other in a true relating.

A co-creative relationship is one in which two souls access more creativity as a result of their loving interaction. An enhanced energy springs forth, enabling both partners to make a greater contribution than either one could have made alone. It is rare and absolutely worth it.

There are three things you must do to bring your commitments into manifestation.

- ✦ Feel all your feelings
- ✦ Tell the microscopic truth
- ✦ Keep your agreements

Holy Prayer

Beloved Mother Father God, I [we] pray for You to bless my [our] heart's desire to live in a committed relationship. Please bless me [us]. Grant me [us] courage of heart to feel all my [our] feelings, to tell

*the truth, and to keep all agreements that I [we] make with myself
[ourselves], with my beloved [one another], and with You, Beloved
God! Amen.*

§ Sacred Action*

It takes two to play this game. If one person wants to have co-
commitment and the other does not, co-commitment is not possible. It is only when both people agree to play that the real intimacy
becomes possible. If you are willing to make the following commitments but your partner is not, it is highly likely that you are in a codependent relationship. If this is the case, examine why you have set up
your life this way.

For the following commitments to work, each person must make
them a priority.

◥ Commitment One

Repeat, work on, and become the following words of commitment: *I commit
myself to full closeness and to clearing up anything within me that stands in the
way. I commit myself to acting from the awareness that I am 100 percent the
source of my reality. I commit myself to my own complete development as an
individual.*

You cannot have ultimate closeness without being fully able to be
separate. In other words, the more fully developed you are as an individual, the more you are able to give and receive love in a relationship.
This stems from owning everything in your life and not making your
life about anyone, or anything, else.

As children many of us saw relationships in which people had to
compromise their individual development in order to maintain the
relationship. Each individual had to get smaller to squeeze into an
ill-fitting box. It is time for you both to agree that individual develop-

---

*The commitments in this sacred action are adapted to our understanding of the work
of Sacred Relationship with permission from Kathlyn and Gay Hendricks and are based
on their work *Conscious Loving: The Journey to Co-Commitment* (New York: Bantam,
1992).

ment in addition to closeness to the other person is important.

In a committed relationship each person takes 100 percent responsibility for his or her life choices, emotions, and actions and for the results each creates. There are no victims in committed relationships. In fact victimhood is impossible when both people are willing to acknowledge that they are the cause of what happens to them. There is little conflict, because neither person plays the accusatory, victim role. With the energy saved through lessened conflict, both people are free to feel deeper love for all beings and express more.

If either person is being less than 100 percent responsible, the ground is ripe for power struggles. Each person will look for the places where the other person is at fault. There will be a tendency to want to diminish the other person to match one's wound.

Space is as important as closeness. Only through taking space for ourselves can we integrate. Taking space may be as simple as a walk or a daily meditation time. In codependence taking space almost always brings up fear. However, in a committed relationship, taking space usually results in more closeness and sharing as each soul deepens individually. The dance of the relationship is renewed and kept lively.

We want intimacy, but often we are afraid of it because of the pain it has brought in times past. When two people agree, they desire closeness; when they state they are willing to clear up their barriers to closeness, intimacy begins.

◄ Commitment Two

Repeat, work on, and become the following words of commitment: *I commit to revealing myself fully in the relationship and to not conceal myself in any way.*

A major opening to love occurs when we shift from concealing to revealing. Most of us learned to hide our wounded selves *and* true selves in order to survive growing up. We then take this into our adult relationships. It costs us, because a close relationship thrives on transparency. Being fully transparent heals the shadow. If your energy is tied up in concealing who you are and how you feel, there is little energy left for intimacy.

❧ Commitment Three

Repeat, work on, and become the following words of commitment: *I commit myself to having a good time in my close relationships.*

As a child how many people did you see around you who were in a state of joy in their relationships? What about right now? As Gay and Kathlyn Hendricks once said, "We feel strongly that a formal commitment to having a good time is necessary to move into a state of co-commitment. We do not know the meaning of life, but we are sure it is not to have a bad time." Why not take a conscious stand for joy in your close relationships?

COMMUNICATION

Communication—the art of sharing openly, kindly, and transparently with another

The limits of my language mean the limits of my world.

LUDWIG WITTGENSTEIN

Conscious communication lives at the heart of Sacred Relationship. One could even say that healthy, honest communication *alone* could heal the world and catapult it directly into the new paradigm.

Barbara Brennan is a healer who left her job at NASA when her third eye spontaneously opened and she had a direct perception of the human energy field, or aura. She went on to write the book *Hands of Light* and open a healing school. When I (Anaiya) studied with her years ago, she said something beautiful and astounding: "when we can directly perceive the energy fields of one another, lying will become impossible!" We will no longer be able to say one thing and think another; we will be transparent to each other. In other words we will be able to share authentically from a place of truth. When we add love and compassion for others to our sharing, how might that change the world?

The word *communication* comes from a Latin verb that means "to share." It also has etymological roots in the Latin word *communis*, meaning "common." Inside the word, we also see two Latin prefixes: *com*, meaning "together," and *uni*, meaning "one." So coded into this word is a new paradigm way of relating—sharing from the experience of our commonality, our essential oneness.

Basically each moment of this precious life comes down to a choice between love and fear. Are we connected to the source of love at any given moment and therefore able to hold others in compassion and oneness? If that is the case, our communication—and our listening—can be spacious, clear, and loving. Or, are we disconnected from Source and tuned in to fear and the human ego's need to get energy from others? When this is the case, our communication can be marked by manipulation, bullying, comparing, judging, and a host of other wounded behaviors. We have all been there! Yet, my friends, the new paradigm calls us to heal our wounded, often violent, ways of communicating.

Imagine this for a moment. You are firmly connected to Earth, held and nourished by Mother Gaia. At the same time, your consciousness is expanded and filled with the divine light of your own soul, of Mother-Father God, the Divine Source. You are secure and loved beyond measure; in fact, you *are* love. Remember, *I Am That*—God lives in you *as you*. Supported by the divine energies of Earth and Sky, you are filled with love. The light rushes up from your feet and also pours down through your crown to unite in your heart, creating a living mandala. Your beloved is connected to Source in the same way. Is there anything you couldn't share with one another? Is there anything that wouldn't be held in compassion? Very likely not.

A Course in Miracles, as received by Helen Schucman, explains that holy Sacred Relationship exists when any two have looked within and found no lack, and therefore choose to join—to create, to share, to extend love.* Communication in this kind of relationship has *no other*

---

*For more on this see *A Course in Miracles*, teachings from Jesus as scribed by Helen Schucman (Mill Valley, Calif.: Foundation for Inner Peace, 1975) or visit www.acim.org.

agenda. Of course, within a holy Sacred Relationship all sorts of human issues can be worked through, by simply using techniques of conscious communication—some of which are offered at the end of this section. The new paradigm that we are creating is rooted in these new ways of communication.

Now, however, let's examine another scenario, which will no doubt be painfully familiar. Yet even as we look at it, let's recognize it as the old paradigm, which is falling away. Imagine this for a moment . . . You feel alone and disconnected from the sacred Earth that nourishes your body, and you feel separate from the Divine Source that nourishes your spirit. You feel a desperate need to get love, and you believe it is *out there* somewhere. You meet another person who feels the same way, and so your frequencies match. You energetically send out little hooks into each other, so you can siphon some energy and feel temporarily loved. All the while, you are afraid that you aren't really good enough and that you will be rejected if the other really knew who you were. So you say one thing, feel another, and use your well-honed bag of tricks to manipulate or bully the other into giving you more energy. You are constantly—and unconsciously—looking for ways to get this feel-good energy from others. You are angry or devastated if others don't speak or behave in a way that makes you feel safe and loved. In short all of your communication comes from a place of fear. Instead of two beautiful mandalas sharing, the energy between you and your partner looks like a tangled web of unhealthy codependence.

Whew! In the old paradigm communication is an ego game filled with fear and judgment. It is crying out for love and healing. When we can untangle from fear-based communication, the new Earth rejoices and opens her radiant heart to us. As our eyes truly open, we will see the field of all possibilities oscillating in light, dancing like sun on water, shimmering in *everything*—we are all atoms at play in the heart of God! The illusion of separation drops away, and our essential oneness is revealed. Here we can communicate with Nature intelligences, with animals, with plants, and with stars. From this place we can share authentically with other humans: we can listen and deeply commune, with or without words.

Holy Prayer

———————✦———————

Beloved Mother Father God, fill me with Your light, Your life, Your presence, so I remember who I am! Help me to choose love instead of fear. Help me to feel and heal the wounded places where I've felt judged, not truly heard, minimalized, or brushed off. Help me to feel and heal the pain that makes me want to manipulate or bully others so I can get love—all in the name of "communication." Please help me to communicate from a place of oneness and shared love. Help me to be so centered that I can listen to my beloved's communication and validate it—even if I don't agree. Help me to practice conscious communication in all my relationships. Thank You! Amen.

ᐳ *Sacred Action*

Conscious communication is like learning a new language: at first it may seem awkward, but with practice it becomes second nature. This new language will become an essential bridge for us to walk across as we move toward our enlightened selves. Make a commitment today to practice this new language.

Marshall Rosenberg, founder of Non-Violent Communication, says that all of our feelings point to basic human needs. When we notice things that bother us, we can express our feelings, discover our underlying need, and make a request. Usually others are happy to help us get our need met. Here is a simple example. I *observe* dirty socks on the couch and I *feel* frustrated, because I have a *need* for order and harmony. I express how I feel, and what I need to the owner of the socks, and make a *request*, avoiding the phrase "You always . . . !" Instead I say, "I feel frustrated because I see dirty socks on the couch. I really need order and harmony in the sitting room, especially at the end of a long day. Would you be willing to put dirty socks in the hamper next time?" Because I have not called the sock owner a stinky slob and, in my frustration, yelled out ten other things that *always* annoy me about him or her, the response to my request will most likely be, "Oh sure—I just forgot. I like order and harmony, too. I will be more mindful next time."

Here is another format for practicing conscious communication that is especially helpful when deeper emotional issues arise. It is called the intentional dialogue, or couple's dialogue. This is one of the most effective forms of communication between persons in a committed love relationship. Be sure to set aside sacred, uninterrupted time for this process when you have something important to communicate.

The intentional dialogue consists of three processes called mirroring, validation, and empathy. Each person in the couple takes a turn, so each has a chance to send and receive.

Mirroring is the process of accurately reflecting back the content of a message from the sending partner. The most common form of mirroring is paraphrasing. A paraphrase is a statement in your own words of what the message your partner sent means to you. It indicates that you are willing to transcend your own thoughts and feelings for the moment and attempt to understand your partner from his or her point of view. Any response made *prior* to mirroring is often an interpretation and may contain a misunderstanding. Mirroring allows your partner to send the message again and permits you to paraphrase until you do understand. "Let me see if I've got that . . ." "I understand you to be saying . . ." "What I heard you say is . . ." are typical beginnings of a respectful mirror. After mirroring, ask, "Did I get it all?" When you have, ask, "Is there more?"

Validation is a communication to the sending partner that the information being received and mirrored makes sense. It indicates that you can see the information from your partner's point of view and can accept that it has validity—it is true for your partner. Validation is a temporary suspension or transcendence of your point of view that allows your partner's experience to have its own reality. Typical validating phrases are: "I can see that . . ." "It makes sense to me that you would think that . . ." "I can understand that . . ." Such phrases convey to your partner that his or her subjective experience is not crazy, that it has its own logic, and that it is a valid way of looking at things. To validate your partner's message does not mean that you agree with his or her point of view or that it reflects your subjective experience. It merely recognizes the fact that in every situation, no *objective* view is possible. In any communication between two persons there are always two points of view, and every report of any experience is an interpretation, which is the *truth* for each person. The processes of mirroring and validation affirm the other person and increase trust and closeness.

Empathy is the process of reflecting or imagining the feelings the sending partner is experiencing about the event or the situation being reported. In this deep level of communication, the listener attempts to recognize, reach in to, and, on some level, experience the emotions of the sending partner. Empathy allows both partners to transcend their separateness and to experience a genuine meeting. Such an experience has remarkable healing power. Typical phrases for empathic communication include "and I can imagine that you might feel . . ." "And when you experience that, I understand you feel . . ."

A dialogue from the sending partner may then sound as follows: "So I hear you to be saying that if I don't look at you when you are talking to me, you think that I am uninterested in what you are saying. I can understand that. It makes sense to me, and I can imagine that you might feel rejected and angry. That must be a terrible feeling."

The intentional dialogue is complete when both partners have had a turn at sending and receiving, so the process is reciprocal.

The next time you feel frustrated with your partner, take a big breath and try the above strategies of conscious communication instead of arguing your own point.

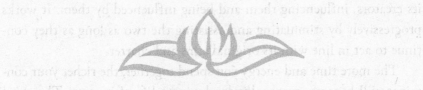

CONTAINER

Container—a crucible that is a sound, safe structure that allows the energies of union to alchemize and form

The greatest of all mysteries is playing out right *now*, and we all have a front row seat. It is no less than the birth of a new kind of human being; one who is united within, containing *all* of the opposites at play in this dance of Creation. This is what the shift in consciousness is about. Here we stand, straddling the old and new paradigms—we are walking over a bridge from separation to oneness. We desire so deeply to be reborn. This birth isn't *only* about the coming of awakened consciousness—but awakening is the foundation upon which this rebirth depends.

These times invite each of us to become a living, breathing, and vibrantly focused hologram of the entire transcendent, immanent Universe. We are invited to live in unity consciousness. And with that comes some serious unlearning. We need to *unlearn* individualization, *unlearn* duality, *unlearn* opposition, and *unlearn* aloneness—because the Universe doesn't operate in this way. The Universe is interdependent, coexisting, and ever changing and expanding—and this is how we shall become.

A container is a shared field, womb, or matrix created by the male and female essences in the partners of any gender combination relationship. This shared field, womb, or matrix safely allows a couple to gestate and birth their relationship into full manifestation. It is made of feelings and commonly held soul purposes, principles, and values that form a loving, intelligent, responsive, and interactive third being in their relating.

It is created when two come together to share their combined energies for a common set of purposes. A true container is greater than the individual sum of its two human parts. It continuously interacts with its creators, influencing them and being influenced by them. It works progressively by stimulating and assisting the two as long as they continue to act in line with its original aims and charter.

The more time and energy you spend together, the richer your container will become, eventually developing a life of its own. The third being of the container is a sort of angel, which strengthens through balance and equality between the partners. Where two beloveds meet in the warmth of love, the third is created, a being of union that knows only love, that responds to only love. It is an actual, living being, a blueprint of union always present. This being waits for the couple to fully resonate with it, because it *is* they themselves in marriage, in union.

The etheric blueprint can become so strong that even if its creators should die, the container would continue to exist and can be contacted centuries later by people prepared to live the path of the original creators. Christ and Magdalene are good examples.

Men with an integrated, healed father quality can sustain a safe, strong, and sound physical, emotional, and spiritual container. When a woman or feminine essence feels this, she can descend into the depths of her femininity and her magnetic, feminine foundation: her womb. She will feel held, nurtured, and safe in a secure environment. She will trust, respect, and admire the masculine essence of her partner.

Women with an integrated, healed mother quality can sustain a safe, strong, and sound physical, emotional, and spiritual container. When a man or masculine essence feels this, he can soften all that is rigid within and let go into the depths of his masculinity and his gentle, patient heart. He will feel received, not judged, and able to fully express all parts of himself. This receptiveness invites him to trust, honor, and treasure the feminine essence of his partner.

In Sacred Relationship this mutual presence, love, and support create a loving container for the combined energies of your shared intent. Your mutual purpose and soul agreements will flow into this safe container and take form in the world. This field is vital in order to maintain the integrity of what is being created, for all processes in creation need a container to bring the formless into form.

The container's purpose is to hold the two together. Its natural quality is magnetic and embracing, gathering all the open and intimate shared moments in lovemaking, commitment, and communication. All the issues that you face and overcome together contribute to the growing strength and power of the container. In return it will influence you and fill you with the courage and the resources to continue to love and be together.

Beloved God is part of the container of sacred union. Allowing and desiring God in your container requires deep emotional intimacy and a personal connection to God-Goddess, which will allow divine love to pour into you as you heal your own barriers to love. The flowering of a Sacred Relationship depends on whether or not you both seal the doors of the relationship and throw away the secret key in your back pocket that represents a convenient exit strategy. When you seal the container of your relationship, you cannot run away; you have to confront what is happening and who you really are. If you close the door, bolt it, turn around, and allow yourself to be in the heat with your partner, you can enter into the mandala of love you have always wished for.

Sealing the doors means no one else is allowed into this sanctum—this haven where only you and the beloved reside and commune. A sacred circle of protection is erected that allows the full unfolding and blooming of love to occur away from prying eyes. The container is a doorway to God for those on the path of Sacred Relationship. For some souls, the container becomes part of God. She becomes the third being in the relationship, dissolving both of your human souls into her. The container reveals more when both are in a state of loving harmonic rhythm. It also manifests at vital crossroads: at the gates of a breakthrough, breakdown, or big soul opening.

Holy Prayer
✦

Beloved Mother Father God, help me [us] create a sound container for my [our] love to bloom and grow in. Help me [us both] feel and release all my [our] obstacles to this. Help me [us] throw away my [our] back door keys and fears so I [we] can commit to my partner [each other] fully, no matter what. Help me [us] burn in the heat of vulnerability, transparency, and love for and with my partner [each other]. Amen.

⑤ Sacred Action Part I

Beloved One, take your time to sanctify your self and your relationship. Are you feeling disruptive energies infiltrating your lives or experiencing the influence of others in an unwanted way? Know that when you and your beloved come together—you are truly a force to be reckoned with. When you come together as one (both internal and external masculine and feminine energies) in your Divine Marriage, you will naturally elevate your union to such a great height that nothing can undo the goodness that you are.

With your partner, create a list of ten of your common aims, values, principles, goals, and soul purposes in coming together in divine relating.

Consider what you have to learn and share with each other, where you realistically feel your relationship can go, and what you both desire and want from each other and the relationship itself.

> *In the face of every cynic and bruised and broken lover—I knew you existed. I am vulnerable and surrendered and helplessly yours. You have rained upon my battlefield with flowers and now the fruit of new life grows within me.*
>
> PERUQUOIS, "EVERY MOMENT IS SACRED"

§ Sacred Action Part II

In this spirit I (Anaiya) wish to share a prayer that birthed within me as I sincerely asked for sacred words to unlock the deepest expressions of love between partners and to invoke the Divine Presence into the sexual act. It is important to recite this prayer *before* coming together in physical intimacy. This sacred action clears the psychic space of any negative, sabotaging energy that may seek to weaken or distract you from the highest forms of union and intimacy. Remember that as we become more sensitive and vulnerable, we will pick up on subtle energies, not only those of our partner, but also those in our environment and community. Therefore, it is important to keep those factors at bay, so you may enter the sacred act of love in a sealed space filled only by the presence of God, your partner, and yourself.

Sit in a cross-legged position opposite your partner with a beautiful straight spine that is elegantly aligned with shoulders over your hips and ears over your shoulders.

Close your eyes and gaze into the blackness just behind your eyelids. Stay in feeling communion with your partner, either by holding hands or by continuing to feel him or her in your energy field.

Taking a breath into the body, bring all your awareness into your belly, your womb/hara, and your yoni/lingam. As you exhale connect with the living Mother Earth underneath you as well as inside of you.

Then breathe her life force up through the body, up through the yoni/

lingam, up through the belly and heart, up through the throat. As you exhale express sound through your breathing.

Take the time to relax in the yoni and let her flower open. Take the time to relax in the lingam feeling the verticality of pure presence.

Let the womb/hara, belly, and second chakra just below the navel open and soften with each breath.

With each inhale drink in the life force of the Mother. With each exhale let the jaw fall open and allow sound to escape through the breath; let it spill out, back down into the Earth. Releasing layers of tension and contraction as you dissolve into the blackness, feeling the sensations in your body as you let go deeper and deeper, as you dissolve.inside. Fully be yourself as you sweetly drink in the Mother's life force in union with the Father.

Women, feel the yoni and throat connected, allow all holding to drop away like grains of sand through your open fingers. Invite and allow this new energy of the loving life force of the Divine Mother as pure feminine spirit into your whole body.

Men, feel the lingam fill with energy and light as the life force moves through your body. Feel yourself as consciousness and presence, and allow the Divine Father to fill your body with light.

When you feel fully connected, imagine your love bed surrounded by rings of purifying flames that do not allow in negative energies such as sex hatred, body hatred, trauma, shadow, or any kind of external sabotaging force. Your love bed is completely protected from negative energy so you can fully experience your divinity. You can imagine these rings of fire as the beautiful violet light of Saint Germain, an Ascended Master of the Violet Flame, who underwent the divinization process and seeks to serve others on the same path.

As you continue to breathe, imagine the two of you before the presence of God, asking, praying for the beloved to possess everything within you: all of your heart, all of your soul, all of your body, and all of your mind. See yourselves surrounded by rings of primordial fire that will protect you from any interference from any source other than the purest love energy of the Divine.

Then . . . . give yourselves absolutely to the process, to God, to each other. Know that the Divine is descending, and know that you are protected. Know you are filled with the highest loving life force to partake in the most ecstatic, tender lovemaking. In doing so you know that you are worshipping the emerging Christ in the other.

Then recite the following prayer.

A Prayer before Union

✦

Beloved Mother Father God, we pray for You to enter into our lovemaking. We pray for You to purify all energies surrounding us, so only the purest love may enter. We ask for You to possess everything within us so we may fully come to know and embody your divinity. Beloved Father, keep all sabotaging energies at bay so we may freely partake in this act of love as love, as light, as truth, so this sexual act may serve the divinization process within us. Beloved Mother, help us to love with all of our bodies so we may serve to open one another's hearts, expand one another's souls, and to beautify one another's bodies and minds. In our deep and humble gratitude we offer this act of love to the six directions so our redemptive love seed may flood the face of the Earth—and so the Divine may enter matter in all and every sentient being. Amen.

Let the dance of union begin.

CREATION

Creation—the action or process of bringing something into existence

Dearest Friend, allow me to lay before you the sacred template of how the priestess and priest harmoniously worked together in ancient times to re-create Heaven on Earth. We believe that we are being invited to work again in this way, to co-create a solution to uplift this world. We are convinced this encoded template contains the answers we have been seeking concerning the environment and our natural reserves.

Over and over again, in all the world's sacred texts, the same formula for Creation appears. The Father is the architect and the Mother is the orchestrator into manifestation. The priest acted on behalf of the divine Father Creator, while the priestess incubated the vision and birthed it into manifestation as a handmaiden of the Mother. By merging with the powers of Heaven and Earth, all that was needed was created. And since we are made in God's image, we are fully equipped to do the same.

The priest clarifies the vision and develops the idea. Because of his wisdom and decisive nature, he knows exactly what is needed. His ego is not involved. With his clear and perceptive mind, he uses the powerful art of invocation to join with the masters and angels and call forth their energies. Once this connection is made, he then accurately projects the desired thoughtform seed into the womb of the priestess. This is either accomplished through intention alone or at times through sexual ritual.

The priestess utilizes her sacred powers of manifestation by holding the vision deep inside her womb, and then she consciously gives shape to it. The seed of the thoughtform is like a child developing in her womb. Through breath, movement, sound, womb magnetics, and intention, she takes the powers that were invoked by the priest and brings them directly *into* herself. She holds the energy of the vision deep inside her being until the time is right. Then she actually steps into the vision and *becomes* it. She merges with the vision.

He is the architect and the engineer. *She* is the orchestrator and nurturer of life. *He* passes her the concept and *she* transmits the feeling aliveness to conjure up the intensity that creates manifested form.

In ancient days the priestesses knew how to wrap energy around themselves. They could intertwine and connect with visions in such a way that they were inseparable from them. The High Priestess in every temple carried the gift of being able to bring into form whatever was needed by those living there. This power can be renewed through Sacred Relationship.

Holy Prayer

✦

Beloved Mother Father God, creator of all spheres and their heavens,
hallowed be thine wholeness. May global peace and balance come now.

May all beings be united as one. Manifest Thy gnosis through us and within us. Guide the way to our divine self-awakening through lessons of self-love and forgiveness. Illuminate the purpose of our self-trials and temptations, so that we may deliver ourselves from the illusion and ego and become divine vessels for creation. For Thine is the way and the truth eternal. Forever and ever. Amen.

⚘ Sacred Action

Look at the way you create, either as a couple or individually, and compare it to the new (but also ancient) paradigm as described above.

Recognize that you are always creating, and your life is an exact reflection of what you create. Creation is your inherent power!

Ask yourself if you are *consciously* creating what you want or if your subconscious mind garbage is creating things you don't want. Let go of blaming others for your life, and choose to take responsibility for *all* of your creations. Clean the mind; become as clear as the priest and priestess. Examine your *beliefs*, for they are the thoughtforms that seed your creations!

Ask yourself the following questions. Do my creations reflect my highest vision? Are my beloved and I creating in a positive, conscious way together? Remember, your union is the highest configuration for boundless creation.

Discuss your reflections with your partner or with the masculine and feminine aspects of your self. You may be reading this quality of love because it is time to create according to the holy purpose within your soul.

Create a positive affirmation to seed and manifest. Write it down and say it daily, with feeling.

DIVINE LOVE

Divine Love—a love that is like or of God

Divine love is the most powerful, pleasurable, beautiful, transformative, and alchemical substance in all the myriad universes. We receive divine love through the invoking of our holy desire, which comes from the depths of our heart as we ask and yearn sincerely, passionately, and whole-heartedly.

Holy desire is an arrow of light piercing your heart. This desire searches every single last part of you, known and unknown. Driving this arrow deep into the home of your heart, your soul, you strike a celestial musical note, igniting a flame that attracts the angels and God herself.

Pure desire is a shining lantern, a lighthouse, a searchlight of love and truth. It is the fuel of holy desire in powerful humility that brings wisdom—Sophia. Longing itself brings the cure.

Divine love is the very substance of God. It is the greatest blessing in Creation that we can ever receive and the greatest love we will ever feel. All we need do to receive it is ask. Divine love makes all things new by helping you to see and feel everything in your soul. What could take many years to heal normally can be done in weeks if you go directly to the cause while holding God's hand and receiving her love. Without divine love you can spend years mentally dealing with the psychological effects of past traumas, piece by piece, and still not be fully, radiantly healed.

We feel divine love first through gentle, kind, and loving feelings, independent of any person. As we heal through our sacred tears, we feel deep peace, joy, gratitude, and celebration. We laugh and cry; waves of ecstasy flow and great humility washes over the soul. Once you walk through this divine door—once divine love is truly tasted—you will always want more, as it is the greatest love one can ever know.

Divine love is infinitely vast, infinitely full, all encompassing, and beyond any mortal understanding. It is so endless and infinite that it can fill every single soul in all universes completely and still keep going and create an infinite number of souls and an infinite number of other universes *and* fill all those souls it has just created with divine love too.

And it can keep going, and going, and going, ad infinitum. And it has done, it is, and it will ever do so. There is no scarcity, no lack in how we are loved perfectly, how we are indeed the essence of divine love. Ask and you shall receive. Tap your heels together three times and wake up to the fact that you are already home.

As our experiences of divine love deepen, we become closer to God and begin to recognize the divine love within our very souls. Divine love becomes so powerful that we are brought to our knees in immense gratitude, ecstasy, and bliss. Our bodies shake and tremble, sweat pours off us, and we are transported. Rumi, Christ, and Magdalene all experienced this resurrection: divine love transformed their human souls forever.

Divine love alchemizes and dissolves the soul you think is "you." The human soul heals and awakens to wholeness in divine love to then birth a new soul, a new you: the Divine Human.

Holy Prayer*

✦

Beloved Mother Father God, creator of my soul, creator of all souls, we are all Your children under Your tender care. We are the greatest of Your creations, the most wonderful of all Your handiwork. I feel that Your will is that I become one with You and never harm myself or any other being. Beloved Father Mother God, please send me Your divine love. Please send me Your holy spirit. I love You with all my heart, all my strength, and all my might. Thank You for Your love and for everything in my life. Amen.

⑤ Sacred Action

Beloved One, have you been feeling disconnected from the source of all love and the lineage of your soul? Do you feel you have lost your way and are wandering around in exile?

Take this time to come into feeling communion with your essence—no matter how desperate you are feeling—and decide now to reach out for comfort, healing, blessing, and love. The Holy Spirit (Divine Feminine/Holy Sophia) is here right now, in this message, waiting for you to call out to her.

*This prayer is adapted from the "Aramaic Lord's Prayer" and the "Prayer for Divine Love" as received from Jesus by James E. Padgett. For more on the divine messages received by James E. Padgett, visit thepadgettmessages.org.

Allow your defenses, your layers of protection and resistance, to drop in this moment. Breathe and let go as you gently humble yourself so you can receive. This is between you and the Holy Sophia, a very private and personal reunion between human and divine. Take this opportunity, Beloved; she is here to receive you.

EMBODIMENT

Embodiment—the representation or expression of energy in a tangible or visible form

Delight in this entire universe
As permeated with divine awareness,
And every area of your body—
Your feet, your face, your shoulders—
made out of divine awareness.

The body of the planet beneath you,
Out beyond the farthest horizons,
The stars and the reaches of space—
All are arising from God-consciousness.

Know this and dissolve into peace.

LORIN ROCHE, *THE RADIANCE SUTRAS*

We are journeying into the greatest of all mysteries, the birth on Earth of embodied human beings that can contain within themselves all of the opposites of this most holy and glorious Universe. Within these bodies we shall experience the deepest love and compassion ever conceivable, all the myriad frequencies of light and sound, and all the galvanic, volcanic powers that manifest this Universe in serenely dynamic, dancing harmony. All of this shall take place, not in some far-flung planet or imaginary astral world, but right here, right now, upon the Earth, and in your body.

This birth is the organic manifestation of a profound, wordless, non-dogmatic understanding of the true self in its true nature as stainless awareness. This birth of awakened consciousness creates human beings that ecstatically open their sacred hearts to invite the deepest penetration of light so enlightenment can happen in the depths of matter itself. This alchemy is so deliciously intent on fulfilling its quest that it continues to pour its celestial frequencies into the bowels of these human beings, into their very cells, which have been covered with the dust of ignorance for so long. These human cells once followed a path of dark obedience to decay, death, grief, and ignorance. But in the core of our divine blueprint, we have this incorruptible longing to be set free and to dance to the orchestration of love.

The real message contained within this Pearl of Wisdom is this— the birth of the Divine Human manifests as an *embodiment,* not just an idea or dream. It is real, it is solid, and it is inevitable. Choose now, Beloved One, to be a living, breathing, vibrant, intensely focused hologram of the whole transcendent immanent Universe! Your very DNA is awakening to its potential and calling you to embody the new human— right here and now.

So how do we take this embodiment of self and expand it into the embodiment of union? The deepest mystical wisdom derived from every form of sacred embodiment is that when we come together in union, we are called to act! Embodied and awakened couples are called to extend out into the world and offer the union of their hearts in a variety of spontaneous and intentional actions.

Embodiment is being present to all your feelings, pleasurable and painful. Embodiment is being present with your body, its aches and its growing pains, its deep bliss and its fulfillment. Embodiment is being present to every sensual movement and sensation in making love and the currents of feeling that weave you together in everyday life. Embodiment allows you to become one with the beloved in feeling, movement, action, and thought.

We cannot hide ourselves away by losing ourselves in the transcendent. If we are torn or separated within, we can become either addicted to the light or lost in matter. Neither of these polarities will serve the Earth at this time; we must pull the light into the dark depths of human existence. In sacred union we must be steadfast and continue to birth ourselves into a couple loving enough to face all that happens, luminous and clear enough to bear the light, and powerful enough to respond in an earthly, embodied way. The holy marriage known as embodiment calls us to be fully light in matter—fully embodied Divine Humans.

> *The universe is here to reveal*
> *Unlimited splendor—*
> *Infinite diversity of expression.*
> *No one can withstand her allure.*
>
> *Adore the colors and shapes*
> *Of her enchantment and know:*
> *The One who permeates it all is a great lover.*
>
> *Deeply relating above and below,*
> *Mortal and immortal, transient and eternal,*
> *Perceive the terrifying beauty.*
> *Be free to suffer and to be thrilled,*
> *To tolerate intolerable ravishment.*
>
> LORIN ROCHE, *THE RADIANCE SUTRAS*

Holy Prayer

✦

Beloved Mother Father God, we ask for the courage to die to our false selves. To die to every separation, every dualistic thought and feeling, every connection to our past, all our karmic confusions of every lifetime—so that we can become liberated, right here, right now! We pray to embody passion, courage, and trust so we may be birthed into our authentic, divine, human selves, so that we can each serve the birth with all of our mind, body, and soul. We pray to become cleared from the false self that keeps us imprisoned and paralyzed in secret ways. Let Your divine will be done. You are the one that gives with

*fathomless mercy and from immeasurable love. Help us to receive all
the goodness You are extending to us now and forevermore. Amen.*

§ *Sacred Action*

Beloved One, are you feeling torn between your transcendent self and
your human personality? Are you experiencing the glorious freedom of
your cosmic being at odds with the weight of pain and responsibility
on Earth? Come, Dearest Friend, let me walk you through the Divine
Marriage: a union of every imaginable form of opposites. Let this experience bring peace to your heart as you embody more of the Great Work.

Imagine your glorious, divine self, standing at an altar. See this one in the most
radiant, luminous form you have ever beheld—smiling, exuberant, beautiful,
kind, and loving. She or he is attending her or his own wedding and stands
waiting for the beloved to appear.

Take your time to really imagine this experience. Feel the butterflies
of excitement, the nervousness, the thrill of joy. Look around you and see
the beauty of the church or temple space, witness the guests, marvel at the
surroundings, and drink in the whole atmosphere.

Your beloved appears at the start of the nave. You can just barely see
the form of the one you love with your whole heart. It is the embodiment of
your human self—the part of you that is weary, broken, and battered from the
onslaught of human and material life. To your divine self, this human is loved
beyond measure. Your divine self feels such a devout fondness for this one's
difficult human journey.

Now, switch your point of view.

Become your human self, which beholds your divine self at the altar,
patiently and lovingly waiting for you. See how his or her heart leaps upon
seeing you and how that warm divine smile fills the space. This one adores you
and cherishes you. You see and feel your divine self and know that is who you
truly are. Yet you also appear as this fully human form walking down the aisle.

Slowly you walk toward the altar. Allow yourself to deeply *feel* all the
emotions that may arise as you take that journey to marry your divine and
human selves.

Continue to switch perspectives. Experience the divine self looking toward the human, seeing the imperfections, seeing the weariness, seeing the illusions and denials—and yet, loving that one so enormously, so perfectly, so absolutely. Then become the human, feeling the divine one's radiance, kindness, patience, and unconditional love. Become drawn toward the altar, pulled by the alchemy of your mutual love.

Go through the whole wedding ceremony, speaking your vows, placing the rings upon your fingers, and signing the wedding certificate. Make it real, make it holy.

As this experience comes to a close, stay connected throughout the whole day, remembering time and time again . . . you are married! That's what makes it real; that's what makes it embodied.

FEELINGS

Feelings—the substance of the soul; the language of the soul, or how the soul communicates to other souls and to the divine

There can be no transforming of darkness into light and of apathy into movement without emotions.

CARL JUNG

Feelings are the very substance of our souls. They are the cause of our pleasures and pains. Most thoughts we have are the effect of unexpressed, unresolved, and unfelt feelings that lie just under the surface. Thoughts are created as a by-product of these feelings and usually as a denial of these feelings. Thoughts do not control you—it is the unresolved and unexplored feelings that do.

When a soul has a deep emotional release and healing, sobbing sweetly devastating tears from the depths of the heart, the mind becomes still, silent, and clear, and thought patterns automatically dissolve. The mind is no longer able to think, and destructive thought patterns once focused around the denial and resistance of these feelings now have the quietude to dissolve.

The mind is no longer in control when we are in a loving, feeling state.

Feelings are waves that marry light into the body. In the process of manifestation the energy of feeling allows pure light to be experienced and to embody in this dimension. Without feeling, thoughts and intentions cannot manifest; they simply create a hardened, electrified outer coating. The soul made of feeling is the master, the mind that expresses thought is the servant.

In the process of manifestation the energy of feeling carries an emotional frequency that allows pure light to actually become embodied in this dimension. As a product only of the mind, thoughts often resist the living field of awakening that is all around us at any given time. When we allow our feelings to unfurl and reveal their interior substance, we enter the process of alchemy—an experience that joins two or more things together to form a single entity.

The peace that lies beyond all understanding comes from deeply integrated feelings, not thoughts. The mind cannot understand feelings, for as soon as you think about a feeling, it becomes a thought. Only through purely experiencing all our feelings nakedly as they are, without analysis, can we enter the depth of the heart and the substance of the soul.

When we let go of the mind and drop down into our hearts, where feeling lives, we can become one with a person, object, circumstance, or living being such as a tree. With feelings, the keys that open the door are vulnerability, expression, breath, and willingness. We have to be able to surrender our little bit of willingness to grace and allow the embodiment to begin. When two people dissolve into a shared feeling at the same time, they lose themselves completely, becoming nothing except the feeling and becoming one instantly.

We unite through feeling. Dissolving into this oneness is true relationship. We all desire to give and receive love in unity with the whole web of life, and it is through the gateway of feeling that we enter the world that God has desired for us.

In this process we learn to let go of what we *think* we need or what we *think* will sustain us. None of these attachments bring us freedom—only chains. Come, Beloved, let us enter the world of feeling—frequencies of union—so that we can not only know ourselves, but enter the bridal chamber and fully fuse with the All, the Absolute, and the Only.

Holy Prayer

✦

Beloved Mother Father God, thank You for the endless opportunities to be love in action. As I take a breath into my heart, I thank You, Mother Father, for your glorious radiance that is shining within and upon me now. Open me, Mother, to my deepest and previously unexplored feelings. Expand me, Father, in my range of emotional frequencies, both human and divine. Grace me with the availability and presence to merge with my feelings and pull from within them the most unspeakable, wordless expressions that can only be transmitted and imbued into one another through feeling. I want all of You, God, as I know You want all of me. I shall live my life as a holy expression of Divine Marriage in every realm of existence that I inhabit. I am Yours, and Yours alone. We are Yours, and Yours alone. It is our pure joy to love You in all of the fathomless expressions and encounters that You playfully send our way every single moment. Amen.

§ Sacred Action

Connect with your feelings, Beloved One. Allow your holy breath to guide you deeper into your heart so you may come into feeling communion with the truth of your desires inside the depth of your being. What are you feeling? How do you wish to communicate your feelings to your beloved?

Connect with all the ways you have been wanting, needing, and desiring the men and women in your life. Honestly look at all the attention you have been trying to get—sexually, intellectually, lovingly—in all aspects of your life. Admit it, you have tried them all.

Now take all this valuable emotional energy and redirect it to the pure desire that lives in your hidden heart . . . the desire for oneness with the Divine. Feel God-Goddess as the one you have been trying to attract all this time. This will uplift your vibration as feelings of love and gratitude carry a high frequency. Let go of the false desire to protect yourself or to keep yourself safe by getting energy and assurance from another human. These feelings are rooted in fear, which carries a low frequency and vibrates more slowly. As we birth the new Earth, we must consciously choose the frequencies of fusion that bring together joy and upliftment. Your soul is luminous, complete, and whole! Feel this, and remember that it is this luminosity that births the Divine Human in yourself *and* the other.

ও Additional Sacred Action:
Sacred Body Awakening Exercise

As you delve into your feelings, allow them to deepen, expand, overwhelm, and take over until you are pure feeling. Whether you are working alone or with your partner, use this practice to connect with your deep sexual nature. It houses a very intimate aspect of your inner child.

Place your fingers, or your partner's fingers, slowly, gently, and lovingly, with conscious attention, at the lips of the yoni or lips of the lingam.

Simply feel the texture, the warmth, the contours, the feeling of the skin. Continue to feel into this as you ask the following questions.

- Has she/he (the yoni/lingam) ever felt respected, appreciated, honored, nurtured, or admired by another?
- Can you remember the feelings of what it felt like? If so, what were they?
- Have you ever respected, appreciated, trusted, honored, nurtured, or admired her/him yourself?
- Does he/she desire to be loved by God and to be filled by God's holy presence?
- Does he/she desire to love with a fullness that encompasses all of your body, heart, and soul?

Continue to ask these deep and internal questions, one by one, slowly, allowing whatever feelings come to arise with each question.

- Does she/he feel safe and secure within you?
- Does she/he feel like she/he can trust?

- Does she/he feel that she/he can open up and be trustworthy?
- What is blocking her/him?

Ask if the lips of the yoni or lingam emotionally feel these layers of distrust. If they do, then simply feel each emotion and sensation. When you are ready, gently send appreciation and praise from your heart, down through your arms, to him/her. Intuitively feel what you wish to share with him/her.

When our sexuality starts to connect with our emerging divinity, it can feel joyous and powerful and at times bittersweet. When we connect with these deeper aspects of our being, we may become acutely aware of how much we have missed these parts of us. There is often a sweet ache of retrieval that squeezes our heart upon reunion. Waves of profound gratitude may wash over us as we embrace our heart's desire to infinitely open up more to God as the fulcrum, the focus, and the center of all. As we surrender to our longing, the alchemy of Sacred Relationship anchors the reality of divinity within our body.

Fear is birthed out of the desire to sustain that which I am comfortable with.

Fear is birthed out of the desire to sustain that which I feel safe with.

Fear is the desire to sustain form as I know it to be.

And now, Beloved, you are to take a step beyond this fear.

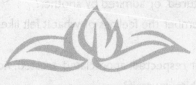

FRIENDSHIP

Friendship—a deep and profound feeling and knowingness of mutual trust, love, and support between oneself and another that has the soul's growth, love, and the divine as its center

Our human love transforms with our own growth in life, with our changes in ideas, desires, affections, and understanding. This love is temporary, subject to change and death; it is not absolute or unending, nor is it full or complete in itself. Human love is the love *within us* that comes from our own heart and soul. It is felt and then expressed primarily for our parents, brothers and sisters, sexual partners, friends, soul companions, children, pets, and Nature. It also includes our self-love, love for our own soul, and loving, intimate sexual exchanges. It is the love we feel when others love us, appreciate us, and are kind to us. This love brings us a sense of unity, enabling us to live happy lives. Without it, there would be no harmony, for only our love for each other can make the Earth a happy and desirable place to be.

Friendship is an important part of partnership and union. It involves loyalty to truth and a higher love. Human friendship is brought into its divine design when both souls involved desire the Divine. Friends are loyal to and united by this common goal. In this deepening, ever-revealing, humbling process, specific feelings of fraternal love arise from walking the path in vulnerability with one's friends. This is soul family, friends of the heart, united through soul yearning and a common aspiration for connection to God. This bond is free, for it is moving toward the infinite, and it is designed to support your soul's growth and the receiving of divine love for each soul.

Friends of the heart have a selfless love for each other, regardless of their own agendas and needs. They will always point out the truth to each other and never collude, for this is an unconditional love that honors the true purpose of the soul and, indeed, the very creation of the soul itself. As friends you support and love each other in truth and free will, regardless of how it may affect you, for you desire for the other what you desire for yourself. You love the other as God loves you and treat your friend as you treat yourself. This human friendship based on the Divine is what God wishes for us, and it leads to more love being created on Earth.

Every true love and authentic soul friendship is a story of unexpected transformation. If we are the same person before and after we loved, that means we have not loved enough.

St. John of the Cross says,

When the friendship is purely spiritual, the love of God grows with it; and the more the soul remembers it, the more it remembers the love of God, and the greater desire it has for God; so that as one grows, the other grows also. For the Spirit of God has this property, that it increases good by adding to it more good inasmuch as there is likeness and conformity between them. But, when this love arises from the vice of sensuality . . . it produces contrary effects; for the more the one grows, the more the other decreases, and the remembrance of it likewise. If that sensual love grows, it will at once be observed that the soul's love of God is becoming colder . . . the love which is born of sensuality ends in sensuality, and that which is of the spirit ends in the spirit of God and causes it to.*

As we deepen in our embodying of the Divine Human and realize how perfectly God loves us, our relationship to God becomes clearer. Friend, Father, Mother, Creator, Beloved—God can be all of these for us, and more. God is always here for us in our humility and desire. Through this love comes a soulful affection for others, which reaches its height within the experience of true friendship. This is brought into its divine design by extending affection, softness, and acceptance to others and to your own soul. The more you love God, the more you love others. This also extends to those you are less familiar with as well as those who may perceive themselves to be your enemies. Sharing affection with your "enemies," being kind to them in their anger or fear toward you, is a sign of this love being perfected. Wherever there is discomfort, there is pain. Wherever there is pain, there is the opportunity for love to bloom once the pain is felt, because all pain shows us where we have not been loving.

This form of friendship gives Sacred Relationship a foundation that extends well beyond this lifetime. It allows us to be totally who we are and have as our goal divine love, something beyond any human partnership. Our human love focuses on the Divine as one power, one heart, and one focus. This silent presence of true support for the deepest part of the soul is priceless and allows the deepest vulnerability to reveal and open the soul into its true nature.

Feeling deep affection for God as a friend, father, or mother is beautiful and brings us closer to the Divine in our own souls. Feeling this

---

*From St. John of the Cross's *Dark Night of the Soul* (Mineola, N.Y.: Dover Publications, 2003), 13.

affection is a vital part of the journey as this closeness means God is seeing us as his child and we are feeling her as our love.

Holy Prayer

✦

Beloved Mother Father God, please bring my soul companions to me now. I receive you, my guardians, guides, soul family, and animal companions. I am ready to allow all the beings that are supporting and guiding me to fully enter my life and to extend their love and joy in the material world as I cultivate and treasure the true meaning of friendship. Please help me walk in life with trust, love, and acceptance for all beings. Beloved God, guide me to be a good and loyal friend. Show me the hidden meaning of friendship and sharing. Thank You. Amen.

✆ Sacred Action

Take a moment to consider who your friends of the heart are. Who are the people who are always honest, open, and there for you? Are you connecting with them regularly? If not, why not? Who are the people who you can always rely on and who you can always connect with intimately, even if you have not spoken to them for years?

Beloved One, have you let go of your old friends and not found new ones yet? Have you forgotten the great importance of sharing together?

Now is the time to reach out to your friends and ask for time together. Even if there are no friends within reach, go inside and recite the holy prayer above. It is time to be part of a circle of friends.

HOLY DESIRE

Holy Desire—a strong, burning, inflamed passion of wanting to have something or wishing for something to happen that comes from your humble heart

Beloved Friend, are you ready to birth the Divine in your own being? Are you ready to risk everything in a sublime adventure that leads to the birth of the beloved in your mind, heart, and all the cells of your body?

This journey takes us straight into the burning magma heart of the Christ consciousness. That flaming heart is the center of the tantric, cosmic Christ, the place where Yeshua and Mary Magdalene birthed a love so complete that it transfigured them both. This love must involve desire and the transfiguration of sexuality, not through repression and not through indulgence, but through the ultimate refinement of holy fire. This love is fueled by the desire to know and worship every level of another's being and by the profound tenderness of total acceptance.

Without this tantric revolution at the heart of the new paradigm, there will be no rebirth. Only the complete blessing and consecration of the body and its desires in holy communion and tantric adoration of one another will create the energies of the Divine Marriage. This holy union means a marriage of both the opposite gender on the *inside* and the opposite gender (or gender essence) on the *outside*. This most magical and holy process can fuse matter and spirit together. Desire is the juice.

So how do we become filled with this burning magma heart? How do we conjure up the heat and passion to fully partake in this fusion? Through desire, my friends, through *holy* desire. The heart of the new paradigm beats only to the rhythm of divine light marrying matter in the cells of your being. This glorious, rapturous love heals the world.

The church denounced desire as sinful out of fear—because desire is the primary catalyst of a deathless love imbued with those very assurances that religion claims it alone can provide. Sexual pleasure was condemned as sinful, so that it was not perceived in its authentic role as a gateway to immortal, transcendent love. In the new paradigm, fear and concepts of sin melt away, and we can once again claim the fire of desire originally planted in our hearts by none other than the Divine.

It is holy desire that ignites your love so that you can complete yourself and your soul's purpose. Holy desire always wants to embrace all aspects of the heart, from the most universal and impersonal to the most deeply intimate and personal, allowing all the possibilities for love in its infinite expressions.

Holy desire is a wanting, an inner burning that propels you, fuels you to keep deepening into the Divine. Holy desire is the deep inner yearning of the soul that can never be stopped. It is passion, passion for the soul, passion for the Divine, passion to fulfill the soul's deepest urges and yearnings. To desire is to live in this passion, always open to following this thread wherever it may appear and wherever it may take you.

Nothing can be achieved without the energy of desire. Desire lies behind every thought, action, and word we utter. It sparks the will to do, to move, to live; it is life in action, linking us to divine will as desire fuels will. Holy desire makes us give our all. It makes us place our very soul at the altar of the Divine, allowing divine will to flow through us unimpeded. For the soul's keenest desire is to be reunited with God in the bridal chamber of the heart, in Sacred Relationship.

If you do not desire, you are not moving toward anything. Desire is the energy that makes all things grow, flower, and bloom. It enables the soul to expand and reach for the infinite and to surrender to the infinite when it comes, despite the fears that may arise. Holy desire never ends, as God never ends. The Universe is always expanding, as is the soul, as is desire. The soul's desire for love, for God, can never be completely fulfilled. It is ongoing.

Holy desire is the beating heart of the soul; it is the life force of the soul, the soul's blood. Without this blood flowing through the soul's veins, we are lifeless, hollow. No matter how enlightened we become, there is always more. In wanting this, and stating this, we let God know we want her, and God can respond.

Want God. Express it every day. Holy desire is the golden thread that connects you and God. The more you amplify the voltage going through this thread, the more God will sit up and take notice and actually send you more through this thread. The only thing that can fulfill a soul's thirst is to drink God, and drink God constantly.

Holy desire leads to love, for holy desire is the love of God expressing itself for no other reason than this is what it must do, for this is its very nature. True desire is unwavering. It is grounded, constant, and consistent.

When the flow of desire is blocked, we start to die. When we forget our passions and allow them to fall by the wayside, we lose a part of ourselves. Death of desire and passion is the death of the soul, a death that only a profound shake-up can then reignite. Holy desire can be an intense force, sensual, powerful, passionate, and overwhelming. This is why many fear it. They fear that once it is released they will not be able to control it as it leads to life force overflowing from within. But when we live in holy desire we cannot be controlled, for we flow in life itself. We can choose when we allow the tap of desire to open, what effects and manifestations it will have, or how we choose to act on any wave of desire flowing through us.

Desire grows through intimacy and intimacy grows through desire. Intimacy, conversing with God and your beloved daily, leads to more opening, more revelation, and more being given. Intimacy leads to the deepest of wounds being exposed if both parties are open to this. Anyone can be intimate in the depths at any moment if you are but willing to be open to this possibility. Wounds may cover desire and intimacy, but they cannot stop you from expressing these qualities in a moment of opening. Being available to this opening is all that it takes.

Holy Prayer

Beloved Mother Father God, I want to birth the Divine in my being. I am ready to risk everything in this sublime adventure that leads to the birth of the beloved—in my mind, heart, and all the cells of my body. I want to experience the tantra of Christ, the great sexual passion that arises when You and I send forth my beloved. And when the beloved stands before me on the outside, I shall love with the whole of myself and be loved back. I want to love passionately and devotedly and bless, bless, bless! I am willing to receive blessing from the beloved too, so that I can be filled with the golden energy of the Divine. Amen.

♪ Sacred Action

Let these words gestate within: *What is it that I desire most, and how far am I willing to go in order to embody and radiate that desire? What fans the flames of the molten magma in my heart?*

The deepest reason to take this tantric path is to be opened up to loving all that is, so deeply and so wildly that you can go through the great death of the false self. When your time comes to be annihilated, you will be ready, because love has brought you to a place inside yourself where you know you are being crushed by love in order to be rebirthed by love, yet again. Pray deeply for this to happen. Embody this flame of desire, which merges you into oneness within and without. In the meantime passionately love what is best and most beautiful in your partner, and passionately love what is best and most beautiful in your self.

HUMILITY

Humility—the noble choice to forgo your own self-importance, feel all your own emotions, and use your influence for the good of others before yourself

Pride makes us artificial, and humility makes us real.
THOMAS MERTON, *NO MAN IS AN ISLAND*

What is true humility? Is it genuinely thinking less of yourself? Is it trying to *sound* less prideful than you actually are? Has humility become the orphaned virtue of our age? Or is it something else—something deeper?

True humility isn't about lowering yourself for the sake of keeping up appearances simply because it's impolite to brag—but to do so for the sake of serving and uplifting others.

Humility is not about feeling small, putting yourself down, and not expressing yourself when truths need to be spoken. People often confuse fear, cowardice, and insecurity with humility. Humility is not feeling inferior to others, bowing to others' verdicts and truths. Humility is true discernment: feeling for yourself what you need to feel on your own unique journey.

Humility is the willingness to look wrong, to feel weak, to make mistakes, to be a fool, and most importantly to grow from all of these parts of ourselves. Humility is being and acting as you really are right *now,* not as you hope to be or want to be in the future. *Just as you are . . . right now.*

The *Oxford American College Dictionary* defines humility as "the quality of having a modest or low view of one's importance," and *humilitas,* the Latin root of the word, means "lowness, or insignificance." But the term was used by Roman culture during the second and fifth centuries CE to mean the noble choice to forgo your status, deploy your resources, or use your influence for the good of others before yourself. The Roman definition of humility goes miles deeper than our culture's comparatively crude use of the word. True humility isn't thinking less of yourself. It's not being outwardly humble, while harboring pride. And it has nothing to do with being weak. True humility is service to others, service to a cause greater than your own personal ambition.

Humility in Sacred Relationship is essential. Without humility, no relationship can grow. It goes hand in hand with mutual acceptance and trust of one another. Sacred Relationship is a union based on augmenting the growth, development, and loving capabilities of the other. In other words, it is based on supporting the flowering of their soul. This means you will confirm, comfort, and complete each person's life-path soul expression. This investment is mutual, although not necessarily alike.

The ultimate level of Sacred Relationship is that of the humble supplicant before the Divine. Humility is an acknowledgement of our placement in the firmament. We human beings are no greater than any other aspect of creation—be it a fly or a pebble—but neither are we less than anything in creation. Rather we are a completely integral part of the whole. Supplication has to do with having gratefulness for and trust in God. As we develop that relationship with an understanding that there is something more than we can fathom with our finite mind, we can connect to the realm that *we come from and return to*—a realm that provides guidance and protection as we traverse the materialistic and prideful world. When we have a clear relationship with that realm, all the losses and challenges of life can encourage humility and spiritual growth.

People who find themselves struggling with anger, bitterness, frustration, and fear at their circumstances so deeply identify with their problems that the problems become their complete focus. This identification spawns an unconscious kind of arrogance that takes pride in being a victim. Ultimately all difficulties in life have a divine purpose. If we can humbly seek that purpose instead of blaming others or blaming God for our losses and difficulties, we will return to wholeness and a state of grace. We have to move beyond these forms of pride or self-importance and trust with a capital *T* the power and magnitude of humility.

Humility is not a state that will come on its own. It takes a particular desire, prayer, and awareness for this grace to descend into your being. Humility is the willingness to feel what you never dared to feel. Humility is the desire to fully feel and release all the painful and pleasurable emotions in you, without punishing, blaming, harming, or judging yourself or others. True humility can be joyful and opening. It brings you closer to others through your vulnerability and transparency. It creates a solid container for intimacy, for deeper lovemaking, for closeness, and for affection.

One of the first tests of a great human being is his or her humility. Humility is one of the most important qualities we all need to develop to become closer to the Divine and closer to our partner. Humility within you and shared with another is the beginning of unity. Humility is the foundation of all true relationships. Humility is complete honesty. It provides all of us with the strongest relationships to our fellow human beings.

Holy Prayer

✦

Beloved Mother Father God, help me to be humble before you today and every day. Help me to be humble to my partner, and help me to be humble toward myself. Help me to be vulnerable and soft and not mask myself behind prideful arrogance. Grant me the blessing of my original innocence and help me to realize and embody this eternal truth: my innocence was and is always here. Amen.

For those who exalt themselves will be humbled, and those who humble themselves will be exalted.

MATTHEW 23:12

♪ Sacred Action

Read through this list and feel those statements that jump out at you.* Then embody the humble person's response—immediately!

- Proud people focus on the failures of others.
- Humble people are overwhelmed with a sense of their own spiritual need.
- Proud people have a critical, fault-finding spirit. They look at everyone else's faults with a microscope, but at their own with a telescope.
- Humble people are compassionate. They forgive much because they know how much they have been forgiven.
- Proud people are self-righteous. They look down on others.
- Humble people esteem all others. They have faith in the potential for good in others.
- Proud people have an independent, self-sufficient spirit.
- Humble people have a dependent spirit. They recognize their need for God. They value gifts from God and from others. They do not resist giving God or others credit for the wisdom or gifts they have received.
- Proud people have to prove that they are right.
- Humble people are willing to yield the right to be right.
- Proud people claim rights. They have a demanding spirit.
- Humble people yield their rights. They have a meek spirit.
- Proud people are self-protective of their time, their rights, and their reputations.
- Humble people are able to love themselves. They do not demand attention or love out of lack or fear. They do not value themselves above others.

---

*This list was adapted from Nancy DeMoss Wolgemuth's "The Heart God Revives," a list that distinguishes what she calls "Proud People" from what she calls "Broken People." More on Nancy DeMoss Wolgemuth's work can be found at www.ReviveOurHearts.com.

- Proud people desire to be served.
- Humble people are motivated to serve others.
- Proud people desire to be successful.
- Humble people are motivated to be faithful and to make others successful.
- Proud people desire self-advancement.
- Humble people desire to promote love and God.
- Proud people have a drive to be recognized and appreciated.
- Humble people recognize that their relationship with God is their primary relationship. They are humble to feelings of unworthiness and sensitive to when they may be becoming arrogant.
- Proud people are wounded when others are promoted and they are overlooked.
- Humble people are eager for others to get credit. They rejoice when others are lifted up. They are humble to their feelings if overlooked and turn to God with these feelings.
- Proud people feel confident in how much they know.
- Humble people know how very much they have to learn.
- Proud people keep others at arm's length.
- Humble people are willing to risk getting close to others and to take the risk of loving intimately.
- Proud people are quick to blame others.
- Humble people accept personal responsibility and can see where they are wrong in a situation.
- Proud people are unapproachable or defensive when criticized.
- Humble people receive criticism with a modest, open spirit.
- Proud people become bitter and resentful when they are wronged. They have emotional temper tantrums. They hold others hostage and are easily offended. They carry grudges and keep a record of other's wrongs.
- Humble people give thanks in all things. They are quick to forgive those that wrong them.
- Proud people find it difficult to share their spiritual need with others.
- Humble people are willing to be open and transparent with others as God directs.

- Proud people tend to deal in generalities when confessing their errors.
- Humble people are able to acknowledge specifics when confessing their errors.
- Proud people are concerned about the consequences of their errors.
- Humble people are grieved over the cause, the root of their errors.
- Proud people wait for the other to come and ask forgiveness when there is a misunderstanding or conflict in a relationship.
- Humble people take the initiative to be reconciled when there is misunderstanding or conflict in relationships. They are loyal to the principles of love and truth first and always and do not allow pride to prevent them from admitting a transgression.
- Proud people compare themselves with others and feel worthy of honor.
- Humble people compare themselves to the holiness of God and feel a desperate need for God's mercy.
- Proud people are blind to their true heart condition.
- Humble people walk in the light. They fully face their true condition and reach out to God from that space.
- Proud people don't think they have anything to repent of.
- Humble people realize they have need of a continual heartfelt attitude of repentance.
- Proud people don't think they need revival, but they are sure that everyone else does.
- Humble people continually sense their need for a fresh encounter with God and for a fresh filling of the Holy Spirit.

INNER CHILD

Inner Child—a person's original or true self, especially when regarded as concealed in adulthood

Often he did not appear to his disciples as himself, but he was found among them as a child.

THE GOSPEL OF JUDAS

Great healers and mystics know that in order to heal the wounds of childhood, you need to go where that child lives—inward—to the spirit and soul of the inner child.

The pain we experience in childhood and from birth makes deep emotional imprints that last throughout our lives, until we decide to feel and heal the wounds and the unmet emotional needs at their core. The unmet need is always for love. Children are totally dependent on their parents and family as their sources of love. As adults we must realize the profound emotional-soulful significance of our inner child. This part of our selves is the one who permits a door to open to deep, caring embrace. Healing our inner child allows the possibility of true intimacy in our adult lives. The inner child may need our love and healing, but it is also the key to our magical connection with the Divine. It is our inner child who, in our early childhood, was deeply connected to God and her angels and guides, who trusted the Divine absolutely, seeing unknown realms as places of adventure.

If our inner child has been wounded, this lives within us into adulthood and leads to sabotaging choices, unhealthy relationships, destructive behavior, and less and less love. As we attempt to make adult decisions, a part of us is constantly trying to protect the inner child by doing the same things we did as a child to protect ourselves—leaving our bodies by escaping into our imaginations, fighting, or running away and hiding. It is almost impossible for the adult self to ever feel completely fulfilled or to be able to completely surrender to divine guidance when the wounded inner child is so busy protecting itself. The protective mechanisms of our childhood become obstacles as adults.

In the mystical traditions, the way you help the adult is by healing the inner child. Many of us try to heal the inner child in adult ways. But in order to reach the child, we must enter the emotional realm and come into feeling communion with the fragmented being within us. When we enter sacred and intimate relationships, it is only a matter of time before this deep inner work rises up for healing in *both* partners. This is natural and applies to all. It does not mean that the relationship is not working. Remember, the depth of intimate love in Sacred Relationship brings up everything that love is not as well.

In essence we have to become both the mother and father to our *own* child. Be aware that when two inner children are relating, complete dysfunction can result! However, when one partner can hold Divine Presence in a loving way, the other partner's inner child has an opportunity to heal. These are the times when we are called to be the parent for our beloved's inner child—as he or she lets go of being the adult and attends to his or her own child's needs for wholeness. This is where our support comes in. We switch and swap until the Great Work is done. As waves of love arise within and without, the inner child responds by coming forward in vulnerability and trust with the willingness to share his or her wounds and desire for wholeness.

Holy Prayer

✦

Beloved Mother Father God, help me connect with my inner child. Guide me to the place within me where my little one is residing. Help me come into feeling communion and deep listening with him or her. Help me to touch the heart of my inner child so I may feel what she or he needs. I know my inner child is crying out to experience wholeness and to feel loved. Help me establish a dialogue with him or her. Please help my inner child to trust again, to play again. Beloved Mother Father God, as my divine parent, guide me as to how I may restore my child back into Your arms. Imbue me with Your parental love and presence, so I may become one and whole with my inner child, now and forever more. Amen.

⑨ Sacred Action

Take the time today to meet and embrace your inner child. Breathe deeply and center yourself. Ask beloved God to assist you in meeting this child self. (Note: your inner child has your birth name, not a later assumed name you may now have.)

Start a conversation and dialogue. Ask him how he feels; ask her what she may need from you.

Hold your inner child on your lap and give him love. Embrace her.

This may take time at first, but the more you make the effort to contact your inner child, the more he or she will come to you, learn to trust you, and eventually integrate within you as part of your flow.

So, Beloved One, I invite you to dedicate one month to your inner child work, honoring the challenges he or she faced upon the Earth as well as his or her emotional needs for love. Your inner child is coming up for healing, and it is because of the presence of love that this gift is here. No matter what it looks or feels like on the outside, the circumstances that you find yourself in are all here as a sign for you to *now* engage in this precious and most rewarding work.

After this piece is done, you will experience years of obstacles being lifted. Many patterns of your life, both inner and outer, will change.

INTEGRITY

Integrity—the quality of being honest, holding values, and having clear moral principles

Discovering and living our integrity is a rite of passage, one we all have to pass through. Almost all of us were raised with the lies of our culture and the additional wounding of our families. We were not shown what is real and true or what integrity is really all about.

Integrity is not based on outward moral judgment of what is right and wrong or society's perception of what is good or bad. Integrity is the way *you* live *your* life according to your heart's moral compass. For example, we do our utmost not to lie. Lying is awkward; it pushes us away from others and makes us feel isolated and guilty deep down. Of course, on occasion, we may find ourselves doing it, but then we can immediately correct it. We also know that being in a relationship where no one is lying makes things work much better.

However, true integrity goes far deeper than not lying, cheating, and stealing. It is an internal, harmonious well-being within you and the whole of creation. Known as Ma'at in Egypt, Pono in Hawaii, Rta in India, the concept of integrity means that we follow divine laws of harmony and goodness, making decisions based on *that*—including what is genuinely right for others. Integrity is intertwined with sovereignty and knowing yourself. It is about making loving choices.

Sometimes we may be pulled toward fitting in and belonging, which requires doing things that don't hold true to our integrity. When we choose integrity over fitting in, we separate from those who live according to traditional social "correctness." Our integrity doesn't have to look like that of the person next to us. How we choose to live and work is different from how others may choose. Integrity does not judge, but quietly goes its own way. We cannot obey the rules of culture or religion in order to feel good about ourselves. This is merely a shame reducer. Healing our deeply held shame and guilt is a vital component to finding integrity. Integrity will help us to check within, find ourselves, and follow *that* awareness to who we truly are and how we desire to live.

Integrity in Sacred Relationship means being completely honest with everything that is happening within you—to be transparent with the other and to keep your word and agreements. Your agreements, your vows to each other and yourselves, are held in your container—the shared energetic field of your relationship. Integrity also means you apologize if you hurt the other and forgive yourself when you make mistakes and stop being yourself. When we live in integrity, we are ourselves all the time—not some of the time, or when it suits us, but all the time, in all situations, with all people. We do not sell ourselves out to fit in or look good or pretend to be something we are not. We do not fake it to make it. We are ourselves, honest and true, even if we fear we may be losing out on an opportunity or are scared we may lose a relationship if we speak the truth. Integrity is the foundation of truth and self love, which is the basis for a loving relationship with others and with God. Without integrity, we are flaccid, wishy-washy, and flaky. Integrity is our backbone, our solid foundation of inner strength and sovereignty that enables us to rise ever higher and manifest more of our soul here on Earth.

Integrity is following your own laws of love, knowing your personal truths and lessons and universal laws of love. Well-known moral laws such as the Ten Commandments and the Yamas and Niyamas of Patanjali's yoga share how to live a moral, clear, and harmonious life. Perhaps the most complete examples of living in this integrity are found in the Egyptian Ma'at, the Laws of the Heart, which show us where we are living without integrity and can gently teach our hearts to live in integrity.

Holy Prayer

————————✦————————

Beloved Mother Father God, I am ready to follow my own moral compass and to let go of the familial and cultural ideals that do not serve my own integrity. Help me to be strong and steadfast, to live in alignment with my own values and standards. Help me to radiate the frequency of who I really am, so all of my creations and relationships reflect the purity of my soul. Amen.

✤ Sacred Action

Bring your journal and pen and pull up a chair and get comfortable, Beloved One. Come into your breath and let's take a look at what is really inside of you waiting to be discovered. As you feel into each question, use your journal to express whatever arises.

- **What do you love doing that you aren't doing?** For your soul's sake, you really *need* to be doing what you love. This isn't a luxury anymore—it's a necessity. The new paradigm is birthed when *you* birth your holy purpose.
- **What type of person would you choose as a life companion?** Forget the mind and its should, can't, won't, or its impossible. Who is in your heart? When you discover who is in your heart, you turn on the forces of manifestation. A whole unlived, abundant life is waiting to rush out of you. By claiming it out loud, you open the gates and give it permission to happen.
- **What feeds your soul? What gives you goose bumps? What makes you fall down to your knees in awe and weep?** Is it

God? The Universe? Starry nights? Nature? Music? Art? It has to be higher than a person, and it must contain the Mystery that surpasses your understanding.

- **How much have you loved?** Count the people. Add them up. *How much* have you loved? Have you loved even when it hurts, even when you thought you couldn't, even when you shouldn't, or when you thought you weren't? If so, you're richer than you feel.

❧ More Self-Inquiry

Self-inquiry can show us clearly, if we are humble, where we are not living in integrity at any given moment. Most of us have done some of the following things. If you state that you have not done them, when you know you have, what do you feel? Can you simply allow yourself to feel the times you have done these things and to really embrace the emotions that created them? This will allow you to come more fully into integrity and therefore more deeply into love.

Recite the following prayer and then allow time for self-inquiry with each of the statements below.

Beloved Mother Father God, I want to grow and know the truth about myself.

- I have not stolen.
- I have not put up hard walls to defend myself.
- I have not pretended to be that which I am not.
- I have not denied myself what I need to nourish myself.
- I have not controlled, manipulated, or invaded others.
- I have not lied to myself or others.
- I have not discussed another's secrets shared with me.
- I have not made promises I did not keep.
- I have not judged or put anyone down.
- I have not lived my life in passionless drudgery.
- I have not stayed silent when my truth needed to be spoken.
- I have not acted small to hide my light.
- I have never betrayed myself or another.

- I have not given responsibility for my actions to anyone or anything else.
- I have not been self-absorbed and ignored the needs of others.
- I have not distrusted or dishonored myself.

LISTENING

Listening—the act of perceiving with the ears; deep receptivity to subtle intuition

Reality can be experienced through the senses only when the mind stops interpreting what it is experiencing. For example, when we listen without the mind defining what the other is saying or interpreting it according to our own lenses of perception, then we truly hear what is being said.

This is the key to all nada yoga, or sound union, summed up beautifully in one mantric sutra—*sravanam mananam nididyasanam*—hear, reflect, realize. When we hear openly, innocently, without judgment or preconception, then we can reflect and take in the energy of what is being heard, whether it is a guide, God, a loved one, the sound of our own heartbeat, or the mantric effect of cars moving on the street speaking to us. In this reflection we realize the essence of what is being heard, and we experience reality as it is—in the power of now.

To be able to do this with another, you must do it with yourself first. For the practice of inner listening can bring us directly home to our divine selves. Attuning to this still, small voice within and really listening to its wisdom is a daily practice that will exponentially expand love in our lives. Patricia Ellsberg, spiritual teacher and coach, has called this the movement from ego to essence, and all it requires is becoming centered and *listening,* often with a journal and pen nearby.* The wisdom, love, and guidance needed to truly listen are all here now—within your divine heart as it

---

*For more on Patricia Ellsberg and her teachings, you can visit patriciaellsberg.net.

connects to Essence, Source, God-Goddess. The practice of true listening strengthens our inner feminine nature because it requires total receptivity. In order to embody sacred union, you must engage in the process of becoming wholly connected with love by listening within. Why? Because this deep inner listening trains you to truly listen to your partner.

How often do we really listen? How many times have you been mentally formulating your own point when the other is speaking? How many times have you absently said "that's nice, dear" to a child's excited chatter, while preoccupied with your own drama? How many times have you idly scrolled through Facebook while your partner told you about his or her day? My friends, these things happen more often than any of us would like to admit! We chronically exchange words without being fully receptive to our beloved's attempt at communication. We chronically fail to truly listen.

One way to correct this is to consciously practice *active* listening, in which we mirror back what our partner said until he or she is satisfied that we understand (see a more in-depth explanation of mirroring on page 190). More often than not, we don't fully realize what our beloved is trying to say, and he or she is left feeling misunderstood in some way. So we must actively engage the faculty of listening as a way to refine our skill. To rephrase what we heard our partner tell us and then ask, "Is that what you are saying?" can seem awkward at first. But it is like learning a new language—a new paradigm language. As we inquire deeper through active listening, we reap the benefit of *really* understanding the speaker—instead of making assumptions that may not be true. For the one speaking, it is deeply nourishing to be fully understood and to feel heard. The Dalai Lama has said, "When you talk, you are only repeating what you already know. But if you listen, you may learn something new."

With practice we will all become really good listeners. We will be able to silence our mental chatter and become truly receptive. We will remain centered in the now, in this moment, where love lives and profound communion is possible.

We must remember that our words hold an emotional tone to them. Often if we really listen to this tone and energy when another is speaking, we can detect where he or she is really coming from and what is really going on. At times this can be at odds with the actual words being spoken. It does not matter so much *what* is being said but *how* it is being said. In listening to this, we can discern and be clear on what is really happening and help the other and ourselves to come into a more authentic and humble space of communication.

Listening means we slow down our minds, bodies, and breaths. Then we can be present to the subtleties. Then we can really feel the deeper meanings of what is being shared; perhaps even feeling a cry for help or attention. Listening means we catch on to the precious nuggets of truth in a conversation and help expand on these jewels to support everyone moving in to a more expanded space.

At times we must listen to our beloved even without exchanging words. Body language is very eloquent. If we are tuned in, slowed down, and present enough, we can listen to the other in total silence. Perhaps a look or a touch is the only thing needed. But we must be aware and listen with our whole being.

The Cosmos speaks to us in every moment. The ancient ones knew this. The Goddess communicates to us through the Earth and all Creation; God nudges our intuition constantly. All the creatures and birds give us signs and messages. Angels whisper in our ears. Are we listening? Everything is alive, everything is connected, and it is all speaking to us when we have eyes to see and ears to hear. The new paradigm world is a magical place and we are an intimate part of it. Listen and awaken, Dear One!

Holy Prayer

✦

Beloved Mother Father God, open my ears and my heart so I may deeply listen. Help me hear Your voice within. Help me hear You speak through my beloved. Help me to silence my ego mind so I am receptive like a clear, calm lake. Help me listen to Your song in the wind and in the voices of the birds and animals. Beloved Mother Father, open my perception to the vastness of Your voice and Presence, open me to the still, small voice within. Thank You. Amen.

ৡ *Sacred Action*

Right now, wherever you are, be still and *listen*. Listen to the external sounds around you. Allow them to drop into the pool of your heart. Watch the ripples fade.

Return to stillness. Listen to your breathing—it is Spirit moving in you.

Now, with a pen and paper, go deeper and listen to your essence. Just listen. Write down what you hear. Whatever you need to know will come.

Practice this daily.

And when with your beloved, commit to listening deeply.

PRAYER

Prayer—a sincere desire and request for help or expression of gratitude to God

The true prayers of a longing soul are more powerful and
will bring the response from the Father, than all the powers
of angels, and spirits and devils combined.

ST. JOHN AS RECEIVED THROUGH JAMES E. PADGETT,
DIVINE LOVE: TRANSFORMING THE SOUL

Prayer is the medium of miracles and one of the most powerful forces that we can connect with as human beings. It enables us to have a direct relationship with the Divine. Through prayer we can personally and intimately ask God to create the most perfect circumstances so that together we can heal whatever needs transforming. Prayer is always answered—though not always in the way we think it will be. Sometimes at the time of impact we may not feel that the situation is perfect—but in hindsight we will see the perfection every time.

Prayer is how the soul communicates with God through pure feeling. Pure feelings, yearnings, deep desires, and fervent aspirations are the language of the soul reaching out to God. This sincerity will *always* be received by God as it is the language of love that God has created for us to be with him-her as our beloved.

Prayers shape the soul, crafting and refining it into essence. In the sublime depths, ecstasies, and heartbreaking moments of genuine prayer, the soul prays wordlessly; the mind knows not, speaks not. Prayer becomes secret and silent, hidden from the minds of all. Prayer is the presence of the gratitude we feel for and the closeness we desire with God. This is when the soul is closer to its secret center.

Prayers are answered when they are no longer intentions, but rather the giving of all of yourself, without reservation, to God. God is willing and ready to help us in our suffering and distresses and has given us the tools to seek her help. There is absolute certainty of this help being given *if* asked for sincerely and *if* we are humble enough to accept the truths shown to us. Only you yourself can prevent God from answering your prayers. By your own choices and actions, by insincere, false, and self-serving prayers, you place yourself in such a soul condition that God would have to violate his own laws to answer your prayers, which he will not do.

Precise prayer is when you direct your desire to God to feel specific emotions, specific parts of your soul, and specific meditations to strengthen your soul. Prayers are answered if they come from humility and soul recognition. Prayers are answered when you desire to follow divine laws and search out what these laws of love are. Prayers are answered more when you make the effort in all areas of your life to heal. God gives us what we need rather than what we erroneously desire born out of the false wisdom of our wounds, needs, and earthly appetites. Choices we make from that false place are out of harmony with love, even if we think they are harmonious with love.

Changing the very nature of the primordial power of desire itself into holy desire for God is another way prayer works well. If you truly come to understand and live the power of prayer, what becomes available to you is a relationship of direct, naked intimacy with the Godhead. With time and practice, this will completely transform your vision of life and all that is possible. In essence you realize that you are unlimited. Every expression and experience of your life also becomes unlimited. When we truly connect in the fiber of our beings with the passion of our minds, the hunger of our hearts, and the yearning from within every cell of our bodies, prayer works well beyond our wildest imagination. Could this be because the Universe is created by a reciprocal relationship, infused at every level by a Divine Presence that longs to communicate with us? Could it be that God is waiting for us to sincerely birth a relationship with him-her and make such communication possible?

The following three relationships interpenetrate each other and can be pursued in your spiritual prayer practice alone or together with your beloved:

The I-Thou Relationship: communing with God as you establish an intimate relationship with the Absolute Only Being. A being that you are related to, made of, made from, in the same way that a drop of water is related to the vast ocean of divine reality.

The I-I Relationship: communing with the soul as you deepen into the deathless, immortal, still, and radiant divine light consciousness that is creating and sustaining your reality at all times.

The I-We Relationship: communing with your sacred task as you deepen your sincere love and kindness toward the whole of Creation.

So, Beloved Friend, the essence of the pearl that you have picked on this day reminds you to turn to prayer—and to not for one moment minimize its impact upon your life. In this Sacred Relationship there are three beings: God, you, and the other. Whether you are in crisis or not, turn to prayer. God is the *assisting force*. God is the *healing force*. God is *happiness and harmony*.

A. H. Almaas is the pen name of A. Hameed Ali, creator of the Diamond Approach to Self-Realization. He has this to say about prayer:

A human being has two faces. Most people know one face, what is called the face of the day. Human beings also have a secret face, the face of the night. The Guest has arrived when the face you face the world with is the face of the night, the face of mystery, magic, and passion. The Secret, the Guest, will not arrive unless everything kneels in prayer to it. Everything has to kneel in prayer—your mind, your heart, your body, your soul, your essence, the Universe, God. Everything has to kneel, ready to be vanished. And you don't pray to it for anything for yourself; you can only pray to it absolutely. You pray only for annihilation. That is the only prayer. The prayer is a passionate love, so passionate in its sweetness that it will burn you up completely.*

Holy Prayer from the Chinook Tribe of Oregon

We call upon the earth, our planet home, with its beautiful depths and soaring heights, its vitality and abundance of life, and together we ask that it teach us and show us the way.

We call upon the mountains, the Cascades and the Olympics, the high green valleys and meadows filled with wild flowers, the snows that never melt, the summits of intense silence, and we ask that they teach us and show us the way.

We call upon the waters that rim the earth, from horizon to horizon, that flow in our rivers and streams, that fall upon our gardens and fields and we ask that they teach us and show us the way.

We call upon the land, which grows our food, the nurturing soil, the fertile fields, and the abundant gardens and orchards, and we ask that they teach us and show us the way.

We call upon the forests, the great trees reaching strongly to the sky with earth in their roots and the heavens in their branches, the fir and the pine and the cedar, and we ask them to teach us and show us the way.

We call upon the creatures of the fields, and forests and the seas, our brothers and sisters, the wolves, and deer, the eagle and dove, the great whales, the dolphins, the beautiful ochre and salmon, who

---

*From A. H. Almaas, "The Only Prayer," in *Diamond Heart Book V* (Boston, Mass.: Shambhala, 2011), 49.

share our northwest home, and we ask them to teach us and show us the way.

We call upon all those who have lived on this Earth, our ancestors and our friends who dreamed the best for future generations and upon whose lives our lives are built, and with thanksgiving we call upon them to teach us and show us the way.

And lastly, we call upon all we behold most sacred, the presence and power of the great spirit of love and truth that flows through all the universe, to be with us, to teach us and show us the way.

⚬ Sacred Action

Start a daily prayer practice. Try it twice daily—upon rising and retiring. If you aren't sure what to say, begin with whatever you are grateful for. Gratitude will lift you beautifully up into prayer.

RAPTURE

Rapture—a feeling of intense pleasure, ecstasy, overflowing joy, and intoxicating bliss that transports us to another world

In the Christian tradition, *rapture* is a term used to describe being carried off, uplifted, transported, or ascended into heaven. It includes a sense of being taken and moved by a higher force into a place like paradise. That is precisely why we have included this word in our alchemical wisdom keys. It is interesting, as well, that the word *rupture* is so similar; it means "to suddenly break open, or burst." And indeed, to feel rapture, a tightly held part of us must rupture.

Rapture is potent bliss, so intense, so powerful, that it can literally knock you out of this world (one often passes out in these deliberately cultivated states). Rapture is a wave that dissolves all things in bliss. This can be activated in soulful lovemaking, in samadhi states of meditation (one pointed immersion in the feelings of bliss and nirvana), in receiving the ecstasies of divine love, and in holy breathing.

In lovemaking rapture brings one into a primordial, authentic, untamed, unaltered beingness. Rapture is a force. In rapture there is little or no physical feeling as you are uplifted into a spontaneous living light of enormous spaciousness and love. It takes you into the unbearable lightness of being, the full power of the ecstatic moment, the nakedly whole power of primordial Shakti fused with living light. It takes you out of your body in full soul orgasm. It transports your consciousness out of the body when you are in oneness with your partner in making love. You leave your body and pass out into bliss through the portal of the womb, where form dissolves back into the embrace of the void. You let go of everything, including time, your mind, and your body, as you experience the formless soul.

Witnessing this rapture and holding your partner when she or he passes out on top of you is quite a loving experience for both!

In samadhi one's third eye opens in deep breathless meditation and floods the whole body and being with potent rivers of drunken bliss. When I (Padma) was in samadhi for fourteen hours a day for two months, I would get up from my sitting meditations to exercise my lungs, which were barely moving. As I went for my walks, I staggered around drunkenly in my samadhic bliss, unable to walk or talk in a "normal," conventional way. Samadhi is the state of Shiva experienced through the brain and pineal gland opening.

In the deep receiving of divine love, joy and laughter bubble forth in an uncontrollable wave that overtakes you. The joy is unformed and boundless, making the body ache with the sheer intensity of this blissful, wondrous, and awesome power. Divine love brings us into the rapture that the angels live in unceasingly, and it is our job to create more space in our bodies and minds to allow this love to become a living, breathing part of us.

So how can we experience rapture? Though it often comes of its own accord, like grace, there are some steps we can take to invite it, particularly in times of challenge.

Step one: breathe

Step two: allow yourself to feel all that you are feeling

Step three: let yourself become liquid

Step four: no matter what, be present with what's inside of you

Step five: accept what is, let go of figuring anything out with the mind

The alchemy inherent in step five often allows a divine reversal to take place: through our breath and presence, the human ego ruptures, leaving us in an altered state of rapture.

There is a saying that *God is closer than our own breath.* Could it be that the Holy Spirit *is* our breath? Could the feminine aspect and expression of God not only be the breath, but also our desire and necessity to breathe? Many traditions, both spiritual and religious, would attest to that truth. Could breathing alone be a key to experiencing rapture? This is for you to find out. It has certainly been our experience.

The following excerpt from Jean-Marie de la Trinite's *Way of the Perfect* describes an experience of rapture.

O my Beloved,

There is no end to the wonders of Thy Love. Just when I think that it is time to stop writing to You because of Thy usual greatness bestowed upon my poor soul and the continuing nature of Our union, You surprise me with greater wonders still.

You awoke me into Your wonders with a remarkable vision of inpouring Power, Majesty and Light that swept into my soul again and again, at least five times in succession, I think.

It was like the Holy Mandala but of an awesome appearance. I was in a Funnel of Power and Light that circled out about me while showing me the interior hub or circle of its center that was a majestic, living, moving Black Light of Life, while the outward cone encircling me and drawing me inward and engulfing me was of a like Living Light of variegated black and white, but the Center was the Living Source and Hub of all of this.

It seemed that I was being swept over and consumed and drawn into thousands upon thousands of Tongues of Black Fire and Living Light in this huge Cone that swept about me and drew me into itself toward its massive, supple and subtle Center, and this Funnel of Glory swept upon me again and again with its myriad, uncountable Tongues of Living Fire, all rained upon me and swept into me at once and again and again, and the Center rose up before me in Majesty.

Then You said to me, in a striking and insistent manner, "I Love you," and my heart was moved to the quick. I replied, "I love You. You Know everything. You Know that I love You." And I fell to rapturous dreams of love until You awoke me for Holy Mass, where Thy Massive Love continued within me, Thy Heart Beating strongly within me and carrying me away into the depths of Love.

I was, as it were, asleep in You, so all encompassing was Thy Divine Presence, and everything, thought, consciousness, desire, knowledge and all things physical a content of You and a continuation of Pure Love that stretched from Thy Heart into all things, such that nothing touched me that was not Thy Most Sacred Heart and the Fire of Love that engulfs me in Your Divine Presence.

I love Thee with the Love Everlasting.

It is I, Thy beloved one, Thy spouse. Amen, Amen, Amen*

Holy Prayer

✦

Beloved Mother Father God, open me to feel your rapture. Help me let go of the constraints and limitations of my mind, so I may open to the great heights of my soul. Help me let go of control and manipulation. I do not want to hold on any longer. Allow me to open, to abandon my fears and distrusts so I may rise in frequency to reflect the joyful light in my soul. I do not need to know anything, release that part of me that imagines I do. Give me the courage to throw back my head with wild abandon as I extend my heart ever more and ever deeper into the mystery of love. For You are the All, the Absolute, and the Only. Amen.

---

*From Jean-Marie de la Trinite's *Way of the Perfect*, Volume Two (Fresh Medows, N.Y.: CreateSpace, 2014), 190–91.

✇ Sacred Action

Unleash your desire to experience rapture. You could try ecstatic dancing, erotic poetry, a pottery class with a dashing facilitator, hiking in Nature, partaking in an extreme sport, or reading mystical prose. Intensify whatever spiritual practice you are doing. Learn something new. Deepen your lovemaking. Pray more passionately.

Additionally you can record the above letter by Jean-Marie de la Trinite and play it back to yourself with an emotive background track while breathing spirit as described below.

✒ Breathing Spirit

Lie down on your back with your knees bent.

Allow your body to soften and relax.

Inhale through your nose and exhale through your mouth. Begin to consciously breathe long and deeply while exploring the inner contemplation— *God is closer than my own breath.*

As your breath comes and goes, begin to deepen your relaxation. You are life itself. Realize in this moment that you are a channel for life. You are a channel of life.

Allow yourself to let go of the need to intellectually understand all this. Simply feel all that you are feeling. What if the greatest secret of the Universe is that your breath connects you with God?

SACRED CONTRIBUTION

Sacred Contribution—the birth of the global citizen and his or her business choices and contributions, which form a foundation for the sharing of his or her sacred gifts and purpose out in the world

This may appear to be an old-fashioned idea: the man provides for his partner and family. Yet it is genetically hardwired in our brains and biological responses. Today many women are providing for their partners. This is because there are two types of men and two types of women. There is a feminine woman and a masculine woman, just as there is a feminine man and masculine man. A feminine woman needs to be with a masculine man, just as a masculine woman needs to be with a feminine man. These polarities are in all intimate relationships. Taking our rightful places and balancing them is of key importance.

The masculine woman can be more of a provider in the relationship, looking after the man financially, or they both can be earning their money. The traditional feminine woman would rely more on her partner to provide for her financially. Yet there is still a balance in the relationship.

Part of a masculine man's basic self-esteem and worth comes from working and providing for himself and his partner. His masculine power needs to be engaged, and he needs to feel useful. If he does not, he will suffer from low self-esteem, leading to loss of virility and depression. If he is earning his income by following his soul purpose, he can help his partner follow her purpose and get paid for it as well by helping her establish her place in the world, become self-sufficient, and boost her growth and independence. He can support her financially while she gets attuned to her soul purpose and begins to manifest it.

Part of the balance is that both people are earning their way by following their soul purpose, not working a job just to cover the bills, no matter how well paid it is. This is soul-eroding work. Today men still have the upper hand in manifesting themselves in the world of work and money, because the hardwired genetic imperative is that women look after their children at home and men go out and "hunt," earning the money for them all. We can honor all these impulses, from the genetic to the soul, through balance and support.

> *Sacred Commerce is the party-cipation of the community in the exchange of products, information, and services that contribute to the revealing of the Divine (i.e. beauty, goodness, and truth) in all, and where spirituality—the return to the Self—is the bottom line. This is participation*

> *that is sourced in celebration and joy (hence p-a-r-t-y . . .*
> *cipation), with choice and responsibility at its core, versus*
> *a participation that is weighted down with duty and*
> *obligation, demands and expectations.*
>
> Ayman Sawaf and Rowan Gabrielle,
> *Sacred Commerce: A Blueprint for a New Humanity*

The need for material equality, a 50/50 split in finances, power, and time in intimate relationships, disappears when we approach relationship from the soul's perspective. We each have our roles to play, and this is where the dance of mutuality and harmony begins. When we each fulfill our roles physically, emotionally, and soulfully, mutuality and agreement occur within our deep masculine and feminine selves.

However, this does not always manifest as a 50/50 split. Sometimes one person will completely take the lead and the other will follow. In a balanced relationship we each take our turn in leading and being led, commanding and being heard, following and trusting, listening and being humble. We each are better than the other at certain things, and when we have defined this in the container of our relationship, we can follow the other's lead, learn from the other, and develop this quality within ourselves.

Intimate relationships are not committee meetings, democracies, parliamentary hearings, or inquiries. Something far bigger is happening: the dance of your souls. The benefits of a 50/50 partnership are a myth and a major reason why we can't cultivate a deeper spiritual, sexual, and emotional union during intimacy. A 50/50 partnership is halfhearted and means that no one is giving 100 percent.

Men: if you want a woman with a dried up spirit, dried up yoni, and bereft womb, then have a 50/50 relationship. That lifestyle will give you a home with dry bones.

Women: if you want a man with a flaccid attitude, limp inspiration, and who talks about yesterday's news in the bedroom, then have a 50/50 relationship.

We are here to *thrive*, Beloved Friend. Let us seek instead a 100/100 relationship—fully present, fully participating, and fully providing. The old paradigm consists of 50/50; the new paradigm is 100/100.

Holy Prayer

Beloved Mother Father God, help me [us] come into alignment and to experience a relationship with myself [ourselves] where I am [we are] fully present, fully participating, and fully providing. Grant me [us] the courage and faith in myself [ourselves] to be born into this new paradigm where I [we] morph and weave with old traditions and new consciousness. Help me [us] to find balance and harmony, which sets in motion an expression of life that thrives and ripples through all time and space, birthing all forms of goodness out into the world. Amen.

Sacred Action

Take a look at your finances and your work, Beloved One. Then ask the following questions. How abundant are you? How do you earn your money? Do you share easily? Do you save? Are you generous? Do you owe money and pay your debts? Are your ways and means of creating financial stability and abundance in alignment with your soul? Do you live off your partner? Do you live off your parents? Do you provide for and support your partner? How do you really feel about that? Are you soulfully content in your work? Is your work in alignment with the new paradigm? Are you *giving to* your community or *taking* from it?

Contemplate your insights—see where you can give more, create balance, and go to the next level of being.

SELF-LOVE

Self-Love—concern, care, and action taken for one's own well-being and happiness

The relationship you are all looking for is the relationship between you and your soul. And everything else is just helpful in that, really. The thing that makes you sad is lack of connection to who you are. Any negative emotion you feel is none other than the loss of your connection, the loss of being tuned in, tapped in with who you are.

ABRAHAM HICKS

In relationships the love we feel and generate between each other brings to the surface all the parts of our very own selves that are not *in love*. Love always brings up its absence. Sacred Relationships reflect our unseen shadows, and we need to have a strong foundation of self-love to embrace and break through the wounds of the past and to love one another authentically. Without this solid foundation, we cannot become divine.

One of the greatest challenges we face is to love ourselves, to love who we are. All you need is love. Accept and love yourself for the fact that you exist, rather than for what you do. Give yourself the space to be yourself, rather than to be what others want or expect you to be.

When you are free to be yourself, you have value and worth. You are listened to and understood. There is no need to wear a mask to please another. You are free to be yourself and to share your emotions with no fear of rejection. In self-love you take the risk of being vulnerable and having open, honest relationships with others. You have no fear of retribution from others if you should make a mistake.

Acceptance is the ultimate initiation. It is because you accept yourself that you want to experience all your own positive and negative emotions, realizing only that you are responsible for your own actions and their effects. This comes back to the practice of reparenting your younger self. Your wounded child was most likely never taught about self-love.

Remember, *you are the cause of all your frustrations*. Once you have sorted out yourself—the cause—the effects take care of themselves.

True self-love is present when we no longer *need* anything from any other person to make us who we are or to make us whole. Unconditional love begins at home, in you. From this foundation all unfolds. If you cannot love yourself, *whom* can you love truly? And how can anyone else love *you* truly? Self-love is the basis for all intimate soulful relationships of every kind. Self-love is the very basis for coming closer to God and closer to your partner. In coming closer to the Divine, we love our own soul more. In truly loving yourself, you will attract your highest potential to you, because *we accept the love we think we deserve.*

Many relationships never really take off because the people do not really love themselves. If each person did love his or her own individual soul, then they could come together freely, fluently, and cohesively. They would be able to love each other truly—without demand, expectation, sentiment, dogma, and without any need to look loving. They would really be able to commune and ignite soulful human potential to a far greater extent than has been possible thus far.

When you do not give yourself unconditional acceptance and self-love, you deny yourself the freedom to be yourself, and live your life to please others. You become dependent on others to make you feel good about yourself, to fill in the holes and emotions you do not dare to feel within yourself. You become rule-bound and perfectionist in seeking to do what society says is right or what you think is expected in order to be accepted or loved by others. You feel misunderstood, not heard, not approved of, and you become defensive. You can become withdrawn and isolated in order to avoid feeling your own self as well as avoiding future rejection and non-approval.

You may believe you are not allowed to make mistakes, becoming your own worst critic, unable to say you are good enough. You tend to set unrealistic, idealistic expectations for yourself, which must first be met in order for you to accept and love yourself. The burden of carrying expectations such as "my partner should be like this" or "I need to be like this so my partner wants to be with me" or "others are doing so well and I am not, oh no!" create a struggle within oneself. Releasing oneself from these expectations is a big step toward being who you really are.

Without having felt and discovered how we do not love ourselves, we give ourselves and our self-knowing away, because we think we *need* to in order to be with another or to fit in to a family or society. Self-love is *the* basis for loving others. Self-love is defined by your actions, what you live into, and what you choose, which all amount to one simple thing—giving yourself what your soul desires most. Then you are truly living the experience of self-love. *Giving yourself what your soul desires most is also what God wants for you.*

True self-love is our center, our real foundation. Love your own soul and the other's soul as God loves you. Once you truly love your own soul, you will feel and understand *how* God loves you.

Holy Prayer

Beloved Mother Father God, please help me love myself as You love me. Help me feel where I still do not love myself. Grant me the courage to take actions today in all my relationships that show I love and care for myself. Amen.

⑤ Sacred Action

Beloved One, do you love yourself in this moment? Do you have fondness and warmth in your heart for you—right now? Are you scared of taking risks? Do you find it hard to trust yourself? Do you follow your heart's desires in your actions in the world? Are you scared of being fully vulnerable? Are you scared of failing and being rejected? Do you have a need for approval? Do you find it hard to forgive yourself or others? Do you blame others? What are the things you would lose if you accepted and loved yourself? What would you gain or recapture? Are you afraid of making mistakes, and if so, how do you protect yourself from making them?

Contemplate your insights . . . Where are you being invited to grow? And then make that growth happen!

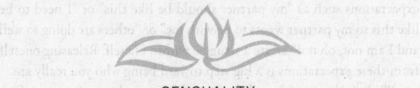

SENSUALITY

Sensuality—the enjoyment, expression, and embodiment of the absolute fulfillment of the senses in conscious union with the Divine

Sensuality is a way of living that we may have temporarily forgotten, but have not lost. It is a delicious, sumptuous feminine expression of delight and a juicy way of living that feels the woven threads of joy between you and your partner. It is a fluid expression of feeling alive, the exquisite, embodied ecstasy of all of life's myriad of pleasures. It is a deep-seated appreciation of being human and a full body inclusive participation in the adventure of life and love. It is how your soul and body move through your worlds and relationships, in play, delight, and appreciation.

Sensuality is not only sexuality, though it does include that expression. Sensuality as a whole is more subtle, more refined, and much more delicate. It is a way of living that is consistently expressing its delight throughout every aspect of life. It is the Goddess in love with all of her creation, living her ecstasy through you, *as* you.

There is a practice known as yab-yum, which is a full body initiation that is designed to connect, then unify each soul with God in all his-her qualities within every level of self. This delightful, deep penetration of love and consciousness (feminine and masculine) is the perfect way to awaken, deepen, and expand your sensuality.

The Sacred Marriage practices that Yeshua and Magdalene experienced were taught in Egypt as *hieros gamos* and in Tibet as yab-yum. This practice was seen as the final stage of enlightenment for both. It is through yab-yum, with an open and inviting womb, that both man and woman can fully heal into presence, giving, and love. In this deepest of all connections possible between a man and a woman, all arises to be transformed. This can only truly be done between two partners who are self-responsible enough to be dedicated and sincere, partners who love each other truly, and are ready to dive further into the depths and climb into the heights with each other spiritually, emotionally, and physically.

In its fullness yab-yum is the union of the Divine and human masculine and feminine within you. It is a journey between two souls that brings together all your mutual sexual energies in every chakra, or energy center, within the body with all the love you feel for your partner and merges sex and soul together with the divine love of Mother-Father

God. To bring human love from the depths of your soul and divine love from Mother-Father God *into the sexual act* is one of the most powerful transformations and healings any human can ever experience. In this way, *no part of the human soul or experience is left out*. All is included. Yab-yum makes us a conduit and a transparent pathway for these energies to meet and merge through the human soul.

The art of yab-yum is the highest aspect of sacred sexuality, and it opens us to a deep awareness of sensuality. Yab-yum is a series of movements, breaths, and infinity loops that merge the great depths of love, sex, soul, and God all together—within two hours! In yab-yum the two lovers generate an energetic vesica piscis that re-creates the beginning of Creation, before opposites appeared.

Yab-yum is the sensual Sacred Marriage of a human being with divinity and the unification of all opposites. The combining of two polarities allows two to work as one, rapidly accelerating and firing consciousness. In this sacred art of union, lovemaking becomes a sacrament, a living ceremony of bliss, love, and power.

Yab-yum is truly a sensual act, which allows and invites one to feel the entirety of the true self and to then connect with the other at the same time. The other is not seen as the goal, as one to be pleased, adapted to, or needed. God Is. Life Is. Sensual expressions and affections between partners will become spacious and emotionally heightened. Feelings of rapture, bliss, and ever increasing waves of ecstasy will begin to spiral into your awareness as you deepen in freedom, openness, and unconditional love. The desires of both souls are met by giving and receiving love freely, by relating to God and one another as the unfathomable depths of being become known to each person. Each partner lives this in care for the other. And yet, one always asks the question: how can I love you more?

The body, sensuality, and sexuality are ways through which we experience duality and separation as well as unity and love. In this union, if there is true harmony and compatibility, your evolution will accelerate exponentially, each of you receiving the deepest lesson and energy you need to complete the wholeness of yourself.

Yab-yum allows the man to regenerate and strengthen himself, manifesting his light bodies into form. Yab-yum allows the woman to embody the Goddess fully as she openly receives the man into her womb, her holy of holies. This sharing of soul blueprints between you and your partner leads to deeper levels of true intimacy, as flesh merges with flesh, and spirit with spirit. This bonding at all levels transcends physical, sexual, and spiritual programming about what we feel relationships are and should be.

Yab-yum creates more than its individual parts in the perfect integration of male and female energies. This reveals a new intelligent force: the Divine Human. Yab-yum returns the visible glory of God's image to the human form. The Divine Child of Mother-Father God lies within you, ready to be birthed as you feel the call. It cannot be birthed into the physical world without both polarities equally unified, both balanced *within* and *with* each other. Then the Divine Human can enter into the physical, allowing Christ to act as the higher self, allowing Christ to inhabit the body. Shekinah, Holy Spirit Mother, acts as the mediator to harmonize and balance the forces.

Divine couples who did this in the past, such as Christ and Magdalene and Padmasambhava and Tsogyal, stand waiting for you, to help guide you into this union of all unions. They show us through yab-yum that form and emptiness, male and female, love and Shakti, God and human, are one. Dzogchen teacher Chögyal Namkhai Norbu teaches us that such couples "also symbolize the union of what are called the 'solar' and 'lunar' energies, the two poles of subtle energy that flow in the subtle energy system of the human body, which is called the 'Inner Mandla'. When negative and positive circuits are joined in a lighting circuit, a lamp can be lit."*

This journey of the beloved is about each individual soul connecting with God. The other partner is a loving support for that. There is a beloved trinity birthing in this sacred alchemy: you, your partner, and God as one.

In yab-yum, yoni and lingam come together so totally that neither yoni nor lingam is felt separately anymore: they become a single unit. Souls come together, and no separation is felt in heart or womb. All of the man moves into all of the woman and is totally received, naturally

---

*From *The Crystal and the Way of Light: Sutra, Tantra and Dzogchen Teachings of Chögyal Namkhai Norbu* compiled and edited by John Shane (Ithaca, N.Y.: Snow Lion Publications, 2000) 120.

and graciously. The woman feels totally safe and trusting in every way and is able open up completely into this. Both the woman and the man feel totally seen in this act. Individual partners become part of a new being that includes both of them, in a new form that is totally each of them, yet neither of them. In this new being there is consciousness, love, and a pure form of feeling. In this there is no goal, doing, or getting, no effort. With the right person, this sensual act will just happen. The technique and method is a way to guide the innate energy of attraction that lies between these two destined lovers.

Holy Prayer

✦

Beloved Mother Father God, please bring me the one I can experience yab-yum with. Please bring forth my holy, tantric companion that will meet me in every realm and dimension. Guide me to expand my sensory awareness, so I may truly love with the whole of my being. Soften and enrich my sensory perception, so I may delight in Your creations. Please help me clear and heal all that stands in the way of me achieving this in this lifetime. Please bring me the people, situations, environments, and healings so I can do this. Thank You! Amen.

🔊 Sacred Action for Finding Your Beloved

If you are not with your true partner, call forth the beloved. Ask. Ask for what you deeply believe you are now ready for. Ask clearly for exactly what you want. Ask for the kind of person who could be with you intellectually, spiritually, and emotionally.

Make a very clear picture in your heart and mind. And ask because you truly want to be infused with the divine energy to do divine work in the world—don't just ask for your own personal satisfaction. That's a wonderful thing, but we're in a world crisis. What we need are people willing to work in the world. Ask for the tremendous infusion of energy and hope and joy that would come from the tantric relationship to help you birth yourself in the world. It's very important to clarify your intention. It's very important to really put your heart on the line with God and sincerely ask.

When you are truly ready, God can introduce you to your tantric partner at a bus stop or coming out of a restaurant. When the time is right, you could be in a cave in the mountains and your tantric partner will walk up to the entrance. You don't even need to be in a very vibrant spiritual world. All you need to do is to create a field around you of wholeness, joy, trust, deep longing, and prayer—and let God do the rest.

❦ Sacred Action for the Ceremony of Yab-Yum

The ceremony of yab-yum includes all parts of you, and the original sacred practice of yab-yum is the height of mastery and union with the true self. Sexual energy becomes sublimated and refined in total sensuality. It becomes a carrier of light to achieve the activation of the new human DNA.

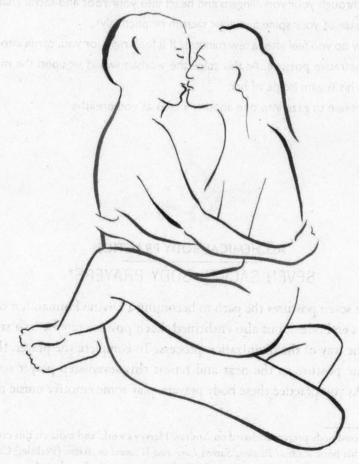

The yab-yum position

Sit cross-legged facing your partner. Or sit in front of a full-length mirror imagining that in looking at your reflection you are your beloved looking at you. See yourself the way the beloved would see you.

Bring your hands together in prayer pose and say "Namaste" to each other from the heart while bowing forward.

Look with love into your partner's eyes, and breathe this love into your heart and yoni/lingam.

Become aware of every sense: sight, sound, taste, touch, and smell.

Start pelvic rocking together in harmony, in rhythm with each other, as the sensory awareness expands and intensifies. The man rocks forward, the woman rocks backward. It can get quite ecstatic. Breathe, give, and receive this energy through your yoni/lingam and heart into your root and sacral chakras (at the base of your spine and your sacrum respectively).

How do you feel after a few minutes? If it feels right for you, come into the fully penetrative posture. At this stage the woman would sit upon the man's lap, with his lingam inside of her.

Continue to gaze into one another's eyes as you breathe . . .

ALCHEMICAL BODY PRACTICE

SEVEN SACRED BODY PRAYERS*

In these seven postures the path to becoming a Divine Human not only becomes embodied, but also enshrined. Each posture represents a stage along the way of the divinization process. To complete the prayer, flow from one posture to the next and repeat this seven-step prayer seven times. As you practice these body prayers, play some emotive music that

---

*These sacred body prayers are based on Andrew Harvey's work, and more on this can be found in his book *Radical Passion: Sacred Love and Wisdom in Action* (Berkeley, Calif.: North Atlantic Books, 2012). You can also find more on his work and his Institute for Sacred Activism at andrewharvey.net.

stirs up your longing and passion for something greater than yourself. My favorite musicians for this kind of process are Hans Zimmer and Lisa Gerrard. Wear comfortable clothing or nothing at all.

⟨ The First Body Prayer

Stand upright, feet hip distance apart, shoulders relaxed.

Lift your arms and reach up for the sky as you ground down with your feet. Do this with great reverence and devotion. This posture represents the lifting up of your whole being to the transcendent divine and the grounding down of your whole being into the embodied divine. Lift your arms up with ecstasy, joy, adoration, and gratitude—as if you are a child, reaching for your divine parent.

Imagine the golden light from the transcendent Father raining down into your being and the rich red light of the embodied Mother rising within you. One energy pours down from the Absolute through your fingers, while the other rushes up from the ground through your feet. They meet in the sacred chalice of your heart. See them spiraling into one another as they merge and coalesce, forming red-golden trails of delight around your heart.

If you feel like moving, please do so.

Stay in this position, reaching and longing, until you begin to *really* feel that you are the living child of the Father-Mother of the eternal light, that you are created from the transcendent Father and the embodied Mother aspects of God. When you realize that this Presence lives in you, *as* you, then with great joy and wonder bring your arms together into prayer position above your head and slowly bring your hands down to your heart.

⟨ The Second Body Prayer

Keep your hands in prayer position at your heart as you stand tall with your eyes closed. This posture represents how the Divine in you blesses, protects, nourishes, celebrates, and adores the Divine in all other sentient beings. Give and receive these divine blessings as you breathe in and out of your heart.

The first two positions powerfully sum up one of the most potent aspects of the divinization process: ask and ye shall receive.

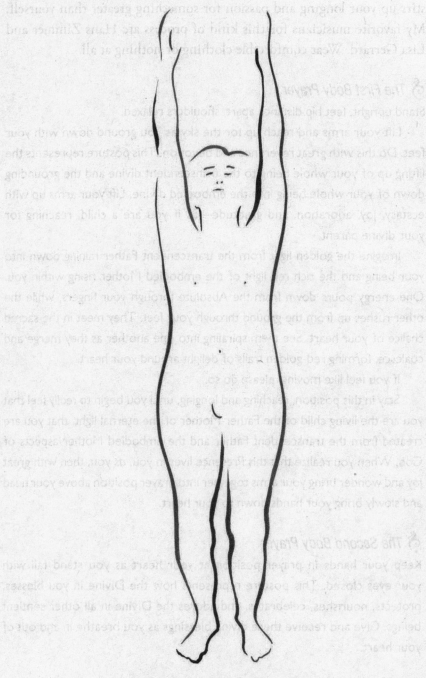

The first sacred body prayer—
standing with arms outstretched

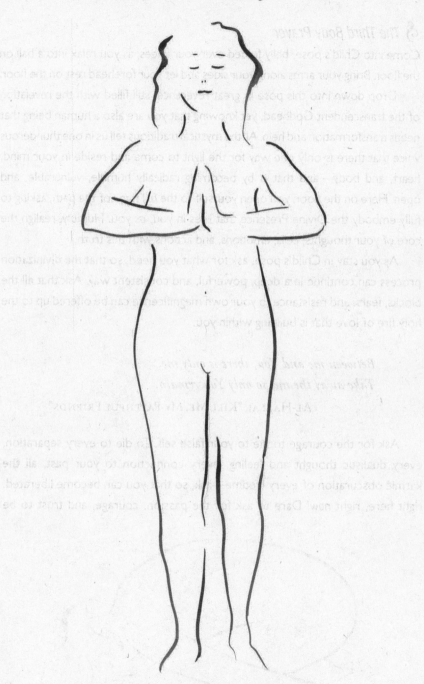

The second sacred body prayer—
standing with hands in prayer position

⑤ *The Third Body Prayer*

Come into Child's pose, belly folded over your knees, as you relax into a ball on the floor. Bring your arms along your sides and let your forehead rest on the floor.

Drop down into this pose in great reverence, still filled with the revelation of the transcendent Godhead, yet knowing that you are also a human being that needs transformation and help. All the mystical traditions tell us in one thunderous voice that there is only one way for the light to come and reside in your mind, heart, and body—and that is by becoming radically humble, vulnerable, and open. Here on the floor, you open yourself to the full rigor of the path, asking to fully embody the Divine Presence that lives in you, *as* you. Humbly, realign the core of your thoughts, cells, emotions, and actions with this truth.

As you stay in Child's pose, ask for what you need, so that the divinization process can continue in a deep, powerful, and consistent way. Ask that all the blocks, fears, and resistance to your own magnificence can be offered up to the holy fire of love that is building within you.

> *Between me and You, there is only me.*
> *Take away the me, so only You remain.*
> Al-Hallaj, "Kill Me, My Faithful Friends"

Ask for the courage to die to your false self. To die to every separation, every dualistic thought and feeling, every connection to your past, all the karmic obscuration of every lifetime—ask, so that you can become liberated, right here, right *now!* Dare to ask for the passion, courage, and trust to be

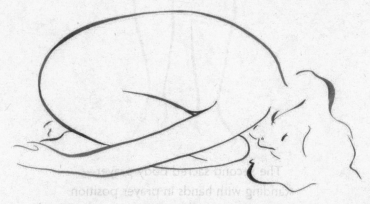

The third sacred body prayer—Child's pose

birthed into your authentic divine-human self, so that you can serve the birth with your full mind, heart, and body. Pray to become cleared from the false self that keeps you imprisoned and paralyzed in secret ways.

Let the divine will be done within you. Allow the One, who gives with fathomless mercy and from immeasurable love, to guide your course. Once you have asked, surrender into the fourth posture.

∮ The Fourth Body Prayer

Surrender into a full frontal prostration, lying face down with your arms outstretched above your head and your legs wide as your whole body comes to rest on the ground. This is the position nuns, monks, sages, and saints take when they offer their heart, body, and mind to the beloved.

In this position inwardly say the following prayer.

> *I am dying unto You. I am leaving behind all my assumptions, all my fears, all my conditioning, all my unworthiness, all my masks, and I am like a bird with extended wings going downward into darkness and not knowing anything. Finally, I am able to trust, with blind love, in the Mystery. Perhaps no one will ever understand, but I will trust.*

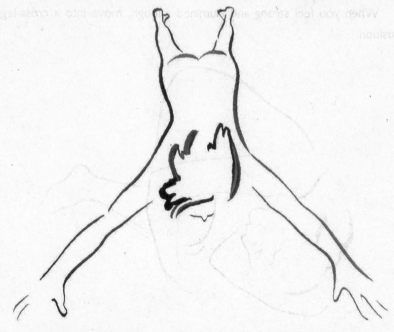

The fourth sacred body prayer—full prostration

That is your prayer as you lie there, sinking down deeper into the abyss. When you eventually reach the bottom, see a pure diamond white light begin to illuminate the darkness. This is the light of resurrection, the light of profound transformation, the light that brings rebirth to every level of your being. This light is exploding softly and coming toward you. It begins to enter every single cell of your being, vibrantly awakening you into your wholly new divine-human self.

Rest in the amazement of this power.

When you are ready, roll onto your right side and move into the fetal position.

§ The Fifth Body Prayer

Lying on your right side, support your head with your right arm and curl your knees in, hugging them with the left arm.

Imagine that you are integrating with great tenderness this astonishing new power of rebirth on every level. Savor each moment of this inevitable birth in your heart, mind, and body. Feel the light in your mind, the love in your heart, and the power within your body. All your desires have become divinized, all your thoughts have become crystal clear, and all of your body has been made beautiful. Every single part of you is transforming into a Divine Human.

When you feel strong and illumined enough, move into a cross-legged position.

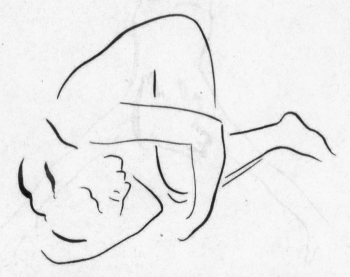

The fifth sacred body prayer—fetal position

ৡ *The Sixth Body Prayer*

Sit cross-legged—like a great royal yogi—with a straight spine and the back of your hands resting on your thighs with thumb and index finger touching.

Witness your total rebirth between Heaven and Earth. Feel that you are a diamond body, radiating divine light in all six directions—East, South, West, North, Above, and Below. Feel that your presence on the Earth alters the entire vibration for all beings. In this moment sit in tremendous gratitude for the grace that is flowing through you into your brothers and sisters of every race, into every species, and into every planet and every universe.

Continue to sit, breathing long and deeply, as you send profound waves of love in every direction.

Once you feel your love fully radiating in all directions, begin to stand up.

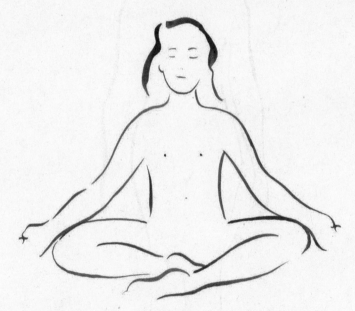

The sixth sacred body prayer—cross-legged posture

ৡ *The Seventh Body Prayer*

Come into Mountain pose, feet grounded and hands at your sides. Stand tall and feel your strength. You are majestic in your fully embodied divine humanity.

Inwardly repeat the prayer

Here I am and I am Yours.

Continue to stand tall as you pray. Muster up as much passionate devotion as you can, and silently affirm that you will continue to stand here, no matter how many ordeals you may have to face.

When you feel ready to move on, inwardly repeat the prayer

I am finally here. I am Yours. Use me.

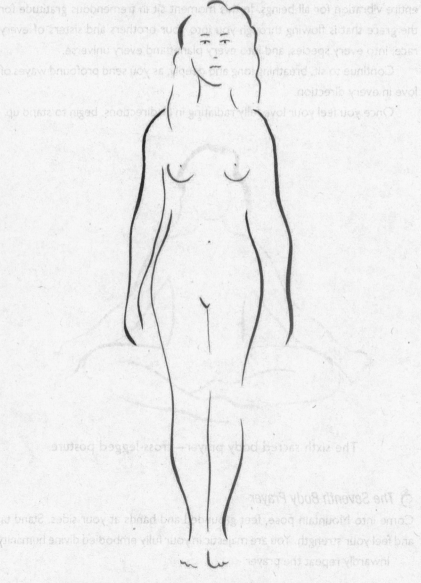

The seventh sacred body prayer—Mountain pose

✦✦✦

Remember to repeat this seven-step prayer seven times. Each time, allow it to imprint itself deeper within you. If you feel called to add this to your daily practice, incredible wisdom will come to you. Because you are working with the body and heart, the Mother will come to you. Waves of *bhakti* (devotion) will infuse you in ever-increasing spirals, until all that is left . . . is love.

SOVEREIGNTY

Sovereignty—independence, self-government, and royal authority to rule all aspects of the true self under the one central pillar composed of love, wisdom, and power

Sovereignty is an inner quality that we first develop and embody through our personal work and then bring into sacred union with a partner. When we are truly sovereign, a royal graciousness inhabits us; the I Am presence of our divine self sits unthreatened upon the throne of the heart. Centered in our *own* sovereignty, we can resist any fearful need to clip another's wings or suppress another's sovereignty. We must be mindful of the ego tricks that might cause us to claim our sovereign state by coercion or out of anger and rebellion; true sovereignty arises out of harmony and inner balance with all things in our world. The divine quality of sovereignty is not wrested from the world by force, despite what power hungry rulers have done for centuries.

Honoring our partner's sovereignty is a gift we give in Sacred Relationship. The more sovereignty we have embodied, the more we can accept in another. True sovereignty is a reciprocal energy—we carry it within and resist any temptation to curtail it in another. When we respect our partner's sovereignty, it often requires us to let go of ego, control, greed, or the wishes of our wounded self. Sovereignty takes us out of codependence in relationship. When we can surrender the fearful voice that says we have to behave a certain way to feel safe and loved, we offer our beloved the gift of accepting his or her sovereignty.

The old tale of Sir Gawain and the Loathly Lady carries a deep teaching about true sovereignty. In the story King Arthur is challenged by the Black Knight who almost takes his life and kingdom. At the last minute the Black Knight gives Arthur a second chance if he can answer the question "What is it that women most desire?" The high king is to return in three days with the answer.

On his way home and back in Camelot he puts the question to every woman he meets, yet he receives a different answer each time. Three days later, with the question still unanswered, Arthur sadly returns to the Black Knight. At the edge of the forest he sees a woman in a red cloak, sitting upon a rock. She tells him she has the answer he seeks. As she looks up at him, her hood falls back and he gasps at her hideous appearance—she has a pig's snout, rheumy eyes, sores on her face, yellowed horse teeth, and a few lank strands of hair. Her body is swollen and misshapen. Yet she offers to save him if he will grant a wish for her. Quickly he agrees. In a surprisingly sweet voice she whispers the answer in his ear, "What all women want is sovereignty—the right to choose their own way." It rings with truth and Arthur knows his kingdom is safe. He turns to go, but she grips his sleeve and reminds him of his part of the bargain. She tells King Arthur that she wishes to marry one of his knights. What can he do but agree? Arthur promises to return with one of his knights the next day. He continues into the dark forest, vanquishes the Black Knight with the correct answer, and returns to Camelot with a heavy heart and a difficult task before him.

One of his sweetest and most innocent young knights, Sir Gawain, volunteers to marry the Loathly Lady. They return with a retinue the following day, and Sir Gawain kneels before the monstrously ugly woman, asking her to be his bride. The other knights are horrified, but Sir Gawain treats her with gentle courtesy. However, that night in the bridal chamber, the Loathly Lady turns into the most beautiful woman Gawain has ever seen! She informs him that by marrying her he has half-released her from a spell, but she will not be completely released until he has answered one question: "Would you rather I was beautiful by night or by day?"

At first he answers "By night, of course, my exquisite bride!" She reminds him that with that answer he has selfishly condemned her to shame, embarrassment, and ridicule in the court all day. "Oh, forgive me," he says contritely. "Then be beautiful by day, my dear."

She becomes indignant at that, and asks why he would want to lie with her at night in such a hideous form. In a flash of compassion and insight Sir Gawain says, "You are a sovereign being, my Lady. You choose." With those words of wisdom, the spell is broken completely.

Recognizing our partner's sovereignty is an unselfish act of love. Sometimes it works like magic to release us from the spell of wounded, conditional, selfish love. By respecting our partner's sovereignty and freedom of expression, we will often be amazed at the depth of love and commitment that rebounds back to us so freely and generously.

Sometimes, however, honoring the other's sovereignty causes us pain as a relationship ends. Yet, as sovereign beings ourselves, would we want to coerce a relationship with someone who wished to be elsewhere? Would this relationship *ever* give us the mutual depth of love we deserve? In such a case we must honor the sovereignty of the other. Then we center ourselves again in love, we choose to trust life and our own divine sovereignty, and we move forward.

We are released from the spell of an unhealthy codependent relationship as we choose to listen to the other and respect his or her sovereignty. We are released from the spell of ego as we let go of the desire for our own pleasure at the expense of another. This changes the old paradigm of control and fear into a new blueprint of unconditional respect and love.

When sovereignty is mutually gifted in Sacred Relationship, we experience deeper love and the freedom to be authentic Divine Humans.

Holy Prayer

✦

Beloved Mother Father God, thank You for planting the seed of royal, gracious sovereignty in my own heart. Help me to recognize and honor this in myself; help me to make good choices and let my divine self rule. Help me to recognize and honor my partner's sovereignty, no matter the outcome. Release me from fear and codependent behavior. Guide my relationship with my beloved so that it shines with a mutual honoring of each other's sovereignty. Help me to also honor sovereignty in all others, including children and animals. Beloved Mother Father God, please help me stand in my sovereignty. Please help me continually remember I am created by You in joy and delight! Help me bring this into all I do and into all my choices. Amen.

♪ Sacred Action

Create a beautiful throne room in your heart. Imagine a throne made of anything you wish: roses, gold, alabaster, or natural rock. Make a throne to match the beauty, dignity, and unique qualities of your own sovereign I Am presence, your divine self.

Now, breathe deeply. See and feel your throne room expand with living light inside your heart. Then invite your divine self to sit upon the throne and claim his or her sovereign power there. The wounded aspects of self may sit on the lap of the divine self for comfort, but they are not in charge anymore. Your I Am presence is sovereign in your heart, and rules with love. Feel the love and sovereignty as a solid strength within you.

Say, "I am a sovereign being, secure in my divine presence."

Notice your royal dignity, your graciousness, your inner peace—your sovereignty.

Take this into the world today.

TRANSPARENCY

Transparency—allowing light (consciousness) to pass through so that objects, feelings, and perceptions can be clearly felt, cognized, and shared

Relationships are crucibles for transformation and growth. You get to see where you really are on your path and where the other is. Each person has strengths and gifts the other will not have, and if both are willing to share and exchange their gifts, both can bloom into wholeness. The key is willingness: what do you value most in a relationship, and what are you prepared to do within the container of a relationship to make it work? What is it worth to you?

We have many different aspects of ourselves. To honor and include them *all* is part of our growth into wholeness and the basis of a transparent, intimate relationship. Highlighting your strengths and weaknesses and being able to transparently discuss where you can both grow and support each other makes a relationship conscious and allows love to flourish with wisdom and self-empowerment.

The following sacred action is a self-inquiry based on an ancient Egyptian way of looking at your self and at life. The different bodies, or lenses of perception, addressed create a multidimensional map showing all aspects of ourselves and the fullness of ourselves as human and as divine. When we work on all of these aspects of our self, we become whole: a Divine Human.

Before we begin, let us create a sacred space by reciting the following holy prayer so we can immerse ourselves into all nine parts of ourselves clearly.

Holy Prayer

✦

Beloved Mother Father God, help me be radically honest about my thoughts, feelings, and motives. Allow the light of consciousness to penetrate my hidden agendas and unspoken feelings. Help me to be brave and to share openly the truth of my inner world with my partner and myself. I do not want to hide behind shadows, lurking around in the unconscious sharing my half-truths. I am ready for full truth. Now, and forevermore. Amen.

ॐ *Sacred Action*

The following internal inquiry can be done by you and your partner. You can practice it alone to start with and then do it face-to-face with your partner. Preferably at the beginning stages of an intimate relationship, ask yourselves these questions from the cool, still center of your being, ideally before you commit long term or even make love, depending on your preferences and goals. However, if you are already in an intimate relationship, it can still be useful to address these questions. Honestly asking yourself these questions about your partner, and then reversing them to ask them about yourself in relation to your partner, can save a lot of heartache and makes your relating conscious from the outset. It would be wise to journal on these. Take your time to feel into the answers.

For each of the bodies, or lenses of perception, below meditate on the questions with transparency first with yourself and then sharing with your partner.

❧ The Physical Body/Senses

Are you physically attracted to this person? Do your bodies fit well together when you hug? Do your bodies curve together nicely in bed? Are your yoni and lingam compatible sizes? Is your partner's body healthy and vital? Does your partner's natural pheromone fragrance smell good to you? Does this person taste good? Does your partner look good to you and look after his or her body? Is that important for you? Does your partner's voice sound good to you or grate on you? Is your partner's general feel, touch, and skin warm, comforting, and inviting? Does your body feel relaxed next to your partner? Does your body feel welcomed, nurtured, and comforted next to this person? Does your body feel excited and alive next to your partner? Does your partner intuitively touch you in ways you enjoy? Is your partner embodied or disembodied?

❧ The World

Is your partner earning enough money to support himself or herself? How does your partner earn money? Do you have to support your partner financially? Do you pay for everything when you both go out together? Do you pay your mutual rent and bills? If so, why? Does your partner spend too much time on the computer, on the phone, and with technology? Is your partner involved in unethical or matrix based jobs? Is this person doing what pays well and not loving it, or is your partner doing what he or she loves, fulfilling soul purpose, and getting paid for that? Is your partner connecting with Gaia in an authentic, grounded, and practical way?

◤ The Spirit

Do you respect this person? Do you admire this person? Is your partner interesting and stimulating? Does your partner inspire you? Is this person intelligent? Does this person have a strong spirit? Can you feel this person when he or she walks into a room? Do you enjoy your partner's company? Is your partner stuck in routine or spontaneous? Is your partner reliable? Is your partner true to his or her word? Is this person present with you in the moment when you speak? Does this person allow unfolding to occur independent of your individual beliefs, opinions, or spiritual paths? Is your partner practical and applied in his or her spirituality? Can your partner freely talk about this? Is this person connected to Nature and animals? Is this person dynamic and engaged? Does this person enjoy life? Does your partner have deep, conscious, and soulfully intimate relationships with friends and others or many superficial ones? Is your partner intuitive?

◤ The Heart

Do you love your partner's physical being, your partner's potential, or your partner's essence? Do you feel love when you are with this person? Do you appreciate your partner? Is your partner devoted to you? Are you devoted to your partner? Does your partner adore you? Do you adore your partner? Do you accept this person? Do you want to be vulnerable with this person? Is this person with you? Do you love just being with this person in silence? Is this person your friend? Do you love this person unconditionally? Is your partner there for you? Does your partner support your heart's expansion and growth? Does your partner kiss you deeply and intuitively in ways you enjoy and ways in which you both meet? Do you feel safe with this person? Can you be fully yourself with this person and express all your heart? Do you have an affectionate companionship? Can you share, support, and nurture this person from your own sense of abundance and completeness? Does your heart sing when you are with this person? Does your partner care for you and look after you? Does your partner forgive you when you make a mistake or hurt him or her? Does this person have a conscience? Is he or she moral, or not? Does this person listen to and follow the heart in action? Is this person generous and giving to you and others? Does this person have good relationships with family? Can your partner sense you and your changing moods and feelings? Does your partner laugh frequently? Is your partner joyful to be around? Is there mutuality in your relating? Is your partner able to cry in front of you? Do you frequently share what you like and love about your partner? What do you value most about the relating between you?

⚐ The Soul

Do you feel that this person really sees and feels your essence? Has this person really dived into the depths of his or her feeling soul? Does your partner have the substance and depth necessary for you to commit to long term? Does your partner have true wisdom and insight in the moment or just knowledge? Does this person really feel gratitude, love, compassion, ecstasy, and his or her own true self? Does this person share this? Does your partner act with the soul's intelligence or the intellect? Is he or she centered in the soul or mind? Can you grow with this person? Does this person have what it takes to hold you and all that you are as well as all that you shall become? Is this person flaky, flighty, and uncommitted? Do you feel you can learn from your partner? Does your partner inspire you to expand? Can you see-feel your partner's pure soul? Is this person humble and deeply desiring to grow as a soul and as a human being in actions, words, and emotions? Can this person walk beside you on your path? Do you feel met as a soul, in your essence? Can this person hold a safe and valid container for the relationship to bloom, despite your differences and ups and downs? Can your partner hold a space for you in which you can grow and totally be and express yourself? Can you be alone when you are together?

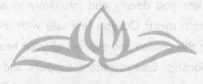

TRUST

Trust—a firm belief in the reliability, truth, or ability of someone or something

If you don't trust your man's capacity to take you open where you want to go spiritually and sexually—more than you trust your own—then you won't open fully with him, nor should you. If he is more committed to attending to his own radiance than yours, and you are more committed to surrendering to your own heart's direction rather than his, you are both still too self-involved to offer your deepest gifts and open without bounds.

DAVID DEIDA, *DEAR LOVER*

When I (Anaiya) first read these words, I knew instantly that they were true, even though actually *experiencing* the reality of them took time. I had never asked myself, *Do I inherently trust this man, more than my own inner masculine?* I mean, come on, our current spiritual trend is to first develop the integrated self—masculine/feminine, light/dark, transcendent/embodied—and *then* go into sacred union, right? Nearly . . . but not quite. There is a vital and essential third step that is often overlooked—and that is where we offer up this integrated self to the high altar of love. Two highly individualized beings cannot experience union. There—I said it! I said the unmentionable. Those who hold on to their sense of self do not and cannot experience union!

Therefore, it seems another element is required, something that I call a *longing,* a divine urge to go beyond individual wholeness into a two-body divine ecstasy. Here the two beings are delighted, overjoyed, and celebratory at the idea of offering up their neat and tidy wholeness and jumping into the wild dance of blurring their edges of self until there is only love. A love that is effulgent, rapturous, and divine. A feeling of unbridled goodness so exquisite that it lights the whole world . . . just as it is intended to.

Here are the steps to reaching that level of trust and love.

Step one: Pray for the healing of self (masculine/feminine, light/dark, transcendent/embodied) into sacred union
Step two: Enjoy, delight in, and integrate the internal sacred union
Step three: Blur the edges of self with another divine/human being,

to go beyond step two into what is unmentionable, unutterable, and yet so very, very realizable

There is no doubt about it, trust needs to be restored in relationship. And how do we do that? By supporting one another to realize we are free, whole, and emerging divine beings. Two of the foundations of love are trust and respect. One way we can trust others more is to feel and affirm their goodness through appreciating them and sharing love and gratitude. But we cannot fully respect, trust, accept, or value the other if we do not respect, love, and value our own self. If we do not love, respect, and trust our own self, we send a message that the other also is not worthy of respect.

In relationships trust tends to be the first thing to go and the last thing to return! Until you are honest with yourself, you will not be able to feel the real cause of your withdrawal of trust, which in fact is your withdrawal of love from a person, event, or situation.

For a woman to experience her deepest sensual bliss and openness, she must trust her lover's masculine direction more than she trusts her own. We are all capable of very deep sexual experiences and very deep trust. Yes, Dear One, I just wrote sex and trust in the same sentence! I have faith that in some wordless way they are utterly intertwined. Our bodies and hearts desire utter ravishment, total surrender, wave upon wave of pleasure, and blissful love. However, usually our sensual experience falls quite short of this.

If you are like most women and men, you know that sex can be better than it usually is. Even if you have not yet experienced it, you intuit a deeper sexual potential, although you may not know exactly how to get there. For most women and men, there are sensual skills to learn and emotional knots to untie. But no matter how skillful or easeful you become, your partner plays a huge role in how fully you will be willing to open sexually, physically, emotionally, and spiritually together.

Deep, ravishing sensuality involves the loving play of masculine and feminine forces. The masculine is consciousness and manifests through the body as presence and direction. The feminine is love-light and manifests through the body as radiance and life force. A sexy masculine person is very present and confident in direction. A sexy feminine person is very radiant and alive with life force. Presence and radiance attract each other and can realize their oneness in the depth of sexual embrace.

In truth masculine and feminine are aspects of the one conscious light that is called by many names including the Divine. For the fullest expression of sensuality, love is also necessary but not completely sufficient. In order for sensuality to become sacred ravishment, conscious light plays as two: one partner embodies the masculine force of consciousness, presence, and purpose, while the other partner embodies the feminine force of love light, radiance, and life force. These days even many loving men and women are afraid to sexually embody these divine expressions. Why?

Every man and woman has both masculine and feminine energies within. Years ago men were forced by social custom to always play the masculine role and women to always play the feminine. Eventually this felt suppressive and limited. So modern-day social custom has evolved to idealize balanced men and women: people who are each supposed to embody both masculine and feminine in psychological wholeness and relational independence. And truly, being whole unto oneself is a sign of psychological health.

But if you cling to psychological wholeness, you won't be willing to relinquish your boundaries of self-sufficiency. Many modern women have worked hard to establish healthy boundaries and actualize their own direction and purpose; relinquishing their own navigation seems dangerous. Yet, if you have a more feminine sexual essence, this trust and sexual surrender is exactly what your deep heart desires. So if you want to open in deep sexual play, you can practice trusting your lover to play the masculine while you play the feminine. Taking the step to relinquish your boundaries in order to realize and express something larger than yourself is a sign of spiritual maturity. To grow beyond mere self-sufficient wholeness, you and your lover can learn to open your boundaries and relinquish sexual autonomy for the sake of two-bodied divine play.

When this is in place, a woman can truly and completely let go, to allow the Divine Feminine of the sacred sexual soul self to express through her. When this occurs during lovemaking, there is often a shuddering, a shaking, a huge pulsing in the yoni and womb. In India this is called Spanda—the sacred tremor of the life force, the pulse of creation and the goal of all tantra. If a woman allows this shuddering, pulsing, and shaking to continue, it will take her deeper into essence. If her partner remains with her at this time in loving connection, touching and nesting within the womb's magnetic fields released during the pulsing, then both can strengthen their bodies of light, entering the womb of creation, or the galactic center.

Many modern men live in fear that at any moment their partner may leave! This gives rise to an unsettled, restless feeling that will eventually lean into the sexual self and eventually the bedroom. This is who we have become. Self-sufficient, self-important, and self-sustained—this is the crisis of our modern Western world. In order for us to actually come back together, to love again, feel again, connect again, we will all have to let go of our perceived importance and rediscover our vulnerability.

> *If you are sexually playing the feminine, you want to be swooned by your lover's unwavering presence, taken beyond all resistance into the overwhelming fullness of love, ravished into bliss. If you are playing the masculine, you want to feel your lover's trust and be attracted into your lover's radiant surrender so that you may give yourself utterly in the ravishment of your lover. As your hearts trust, your boundaries are relinquished, and masculine and feminine open—sometimes savagely, sometimes sublimely—as one conscious light.*
>
> DAVID DEIDA, *BLUE TRUTH: A SPIRITUAL GUIDE TO LIFE AND DEATH AND LOVE AND SEX*

Holy Prayer

---✦---

Beloved Mother Father God, creator of my [our] soul[s], please help me [us] to trust in my partner [one another] and the evolutionary force of this rebirth. Help me [us] to dig deeper into my [our] surrender and ability to let go, knowing that You will catch me [us]. Help me [us] to remember that there is nowhere to go, but to fall back into You—my [our] beloved God. Help me [us] to dissolve the patterns of fear that lead me [us] to distrust my partner [one another]. Help me [us] to love and trust so deeply that my partner and I [we] light the whole world with our effulgent goodness. Grace me [us] the courage to trust, the surety of my [our] faith, and the joy of my [our] goodness so that more and more love can flow through me [us] out into the world. Amen.

♪ Sacred Action

In your personal life you must get very, very clear now. You must address the needs of your heart, and listen to what your soul is asking of you.

Listen and act on what you are being shown in the very far reaches of your heart as you read these words on trust. Now is not a time when you can settle for scraps—a mediocre existence or the kind of relationship that runs on lower forms of energy. I invite you to make a stand and release all that no longer serves your precious evolution and holy purpose toward humanity and Earth. Cherish your self; trust that life has brought you to exactly the right place—here and now. Trust that when you drop the skin of self-protection and control, love already has you in its eternal arms.

Women, ask yourselves the following questions. Do you have faith in your partner's masculine direction—more than your own? If not, can you let go and find that faith? If the deep inherent wisdom within you whispers *no*, ask yourself these questions. Would you continue to stay in this situation/relationship/location/pattern if you believed that more was possible? If you believed that what you came here to give would make a vital difference to the world?

Men, ask yourselves the following questions. Do you trust your own masculine direction more than your partner's? Do you feel emasculated by your partner's masculine direction? Are you willing to step into your own masculine direction in a loving conscious way? What would you do now if you thought that Sacred Relationship would truly serve the full awakening of your soul? What would you do differently if you believed, deep in your soul, that you deserve to give all your precious gifts, talents, energy, and love in union with another? Are you willing to trust life to take you there?

ALCHEMICAL BODY PRACTICE

TAKING THE WAR OUT OF MAN

"Taking the War out of Man" is an ancient process from the days of the Temple, when the Goddess lived in the hearts and souls of men and women. Priestesses undertook this deep and skillful healing to facilitate the return of men in body, mind, and spirit after a long, drawn-out war. The men were invited to pass through the temple doors before returning home to their wives and children. This was a natural and normal way of life. The priestesses were regarded as holy women even in their sexuality, and they were known as handmaidens of the Mother; they were not seen as a threat. The men left the nightmare of the battlefield and passed through the temple doors with the full permission and deep gratitude of their families, who knew this work was essential, sacred, and of the highest integrity.

Inside the temple walls, a priestess would bathe, soothe, comfort, and anoint all of a man's wounds—physical, psychological, emotional, and spiritual. As she worked, she would expand her magnetic field to absorb the man's wounded energy, literally drawing the effects of war—all fragmented memories, fearful thoughts, and hidden traumas—out of his system. Thus, through the power and purity of her energy field and her feminine womb, she would gently and tenderly love him back into wholeness.

This profound healing was gifted to man not because the priestess took on his wounds, but because she could transmute his suffering with the purity and power of her radiance. The luminosity of these temple prostitutes was of the highest light, not because they were gifted or special, though they were trained, but because they loved with all of their bodies. Their connection to the Mother was unsullied and pure, and hence their beings were incorruptible and deeply comforting.

We would like to share with you this ancient practice, as we believe it to be an innate feminine ability that has not been lost. We all have a connection to the Divine Feminine power, which can be easily reactivated.

Keep in mind that consciousness has expanded since the days of the temple and now this practice is not strictly limited to a man and a woman; it simply relates to the inner masculine and feminine aspects of our being. The process can easily be used by same gender couples and also by men with a strong feminine essence who feel inclined to heal any out of balance masculine energy within a female partner or a friend. Merely for the sake of simplicity, we will use the term *priestess* for those channeling their inner feminine energy and *man* for those receiving the healing.

◥ The Practice

As the priestess, you are first required to connect with your deepest essence, both as a human and as a handmaiden of the Divine.

Take several slow, deep breaths and feel the radiance of your inner body expand in light. Let it vibrate throughout your energy field. Feel your heart fill with this Divine Presence.

Next, offer up your full heart to your beloved. This is the one whom you love with all of your soul. Whether or not the beloved is personally known to you doesn't matter—just connect to the love and the calling of your soul. Ask for the blessing of the Holy Spirit, using any words or images of your choice. Ask that this blessing will permeate your being, your partner, and the sacred space of this holy work.

When you feel connected, create a sacred temple space in your bathroom and bedroom; you want an environment that is warm, comforting, healing, and safe. Make sure that all electrical devices are kept to a minimum and the WiFi has been turned off.

Run a bath and keep the room minimally lit with only a few candles. Sprinkle sea salts, oils, and healing essences into the running water. As your hands swirl the water, imbue it with love and healing.

Guide the man to the bath while holding a sacred space between you. This isn't a time for talking or behaving in your normal way—this is a time for holiness and for grace to descend. As he slides into the water, play some soothing and spacious music to help him destress and unwind. Another beautiful suggestion is to gently sing or hum. Your human voice carries the highest healing resonance. You are not necessarily singing *to* him, but rather *for* him. You are creating sounds that bless and comfort him, while letting him know that you are there, within reach and aware of him constantly.

After he has soaked you may wash him, if he hasn't already done this himself. Then he will get out of the bath and you can dry him off with a generous warm towel. Gently lead him to the next sacred space and offer him some simple, comfy clothes like a sarong or yoga pants. He does not need to be naked, but if it's warm enough—why not?

Invite him to stand with his arms by his sides, palms open, eyes closed. Be sure he feels secure, stable, and comfortable. With appropriate music playing, channel the love in your heart to the palms of your hands. Then slowly and tenderly stroke his face, his neck, his arms, his hands, his chest, his torso, his back, his legs, and his feet, from top to bottom. Make sure that your strokes are long and meticulous, not short and frenzied. They need to be long and deep, as you imagine yourself drawing particles of stress and fragmentation to the surface, like iron filings being drawn to a magnet. Long, slow, and purposeful is the energy of this work. Your hands will collect the fractured energy, but not absorb it. When you have completely stroked his whole body—from head to hands to feet—you may shake off the negative "iron filings" toward the earth with the intention that they return back to Source.

Now, guide the man to lie down on his back, with his head resting between your legs. You can support yourself against a wall or use the head board of your bed. You will need support as you gently cup the back of his head in your hands. Softly encourage him to let go and surrender the weight of his head. This takes time and occasional delicate reminders.

When he has given you his full weight, begin to slowly massage the back of his head where it joins the neck. This is the part of the brain that is the most ancient, the area called the "reptilian brain." It is here that we find the amygdalae, two almond-shaped masses of gray matter responsible for the storage of memories associated with highly emotional events. Use the pads of your fingers, rather than the nails as you slowly rub this region. Imagine and intend for an outpouring of love through your fingers into the density of this part of the brain. Again return to the vision of particles and fragments of

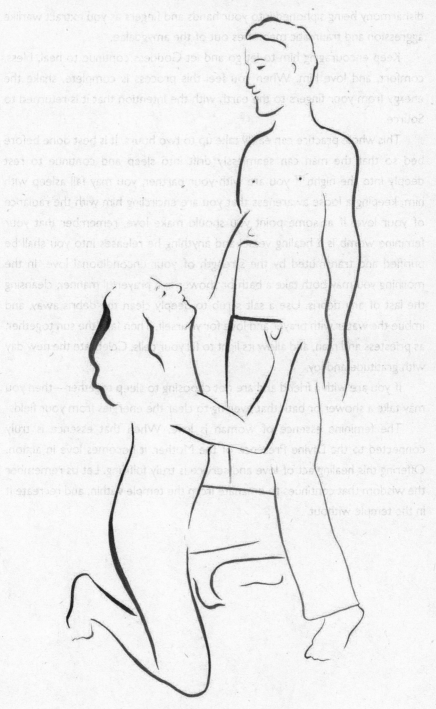

Taking the war out of man

disharmony being siphoned into your hands and fingers as you extract warlike aggression and traumatic memories out of the amygdalae.

Keep encouraging him to let go and let Goddess continue to heal, bless, comfort, and love him. When you feel this process is complete, shake the energy from your fingers to the earth with the intention that it is returned to Source.

This whole practice can easily take up to two hours. It is best done before bed so that the man can seamlessly drift into sleep and continue to rest deeply into the night. If you are with your partner, you may fall asleep with him, keeping a loose awareness that you are encircling him with the radiance of your love. If at some point you should make love, remember that your feminine womb is a healing vessel and anything he releases into you shall be purified and transmuted by the strength of your unconditional love. In the morning you may both take a bath or shower in a prayerful manner, cleansing the last of any debris. Use a salt scrub to deeply clean the debris away, and imbue the water with prayer and love for yourself. Then face the sun together, as priestess and man, and allow its light to fill your cells. Celebrate the new day with gratitude and joy.

If you are with a friend and are not choosing to sleep together—then you may take a shower or bath that evening to clear the energies from your field.

The feminine essence of woman is love. When that essence is truly connected to the Divine Presence of the Mother, it becomes love in action. Offering this healing act of love and service is truly fulfilling. Let us remember the wisdom that continues to emanate from the temple within, and recreate it in the temple without.

PARTING WORDS
FROM ANAIYA

Beloved Friend, as we come to a close with this revelatory ancient new wisdom, let us crystallize what we are being invited into. I encourage you to be clear about what you are calling in and/or settling for. I believe the quality of your relationships determines the quality of the birthing force the Divine Feminine demands from us now—as she organizes her creation to be able to withstand, integrate, and ground the changes she is already making upon the face of this Earth.

I believe without this quality—the pure, conscious, fully present relationship—there will be no real and genuine love or intimacy among humans. The whole species will go into chaos, and there will be no leap of evolutionary change noted within history—because we simply won't be here anymore. The Great Mother would transform this planet, without us.

So, with great sobriety and humility, let us look once again at the staggering adventure that awaits us.

Embarking on a Sacred Relationship is a prayer and journey with someone who is willing to go through this enormously strange experience of uncovering his or her own divine humanity *with you*, while allowing you to blossom completely as well. This level of relationship has to be treated with the greatest delicacy and reverence—because everything is at stake. Either you will cling to your ego, resist, and eventually separate or melt in deep trust, allow, and let go. That is why Sacred Relationship is one of the most radical agents of transformation designed to reach the very core of your life as well as being extremely terrifying, sublime, and exciting.

What is trying to be born through us is a Divine Humanity that is one with its sacred Source. When that humanity is here, the days of the hierarchies that try to keep us enslaved to our lower nature by dominating us with blame and shame will be over. No one and no thing will be able to control you, because you will be liberated in the sacred core of your life. And that is, of course, at the same time why Sacred Relationship is so dangerous and *the key* to this great and wild new birth.

The greatest longing of humanity is to be one, at the most primordial level, with another whom you recognize as being an emissary and ambassador of the Divine and who recognizes you as holy and sacred on every level and in every aspect of your own being. And this connection can never be satisfied by someone who is operating falsely, even if it is in the name of "Sacred Relationship," because all he or she is doing is feasting his or her ego, and he or she will never come into the dimension of union that is the great gift of Sacred Relationship—everything we long for and the very reason for incarnation.

We are being invited to unlock the divine-bliss energies in the body, overseen by the sacred heart, as we enter into a new and unparalleled sacred transformation. This high alchemy produces a body that has become ensouled and a soul that has become embodied.

This is the Mystery the Great Mother needs us to embrace to transform this world.

MAY THE GRACE OF THIS WISDOM
BE WITH YOU ALWAYS,
ANAIYA SOPHIA

PARTING WORDS
FROM PADMA

Sacred Relationship is a dance between two individuals and their togetherness as a couple. One part of your Sacred Relationship is knowing what fulfills you, what your deepest desires are, what your lessons are in life, and how to heal them. This sovereignty is a dance of inclusion with the other: How do they fit into your own soul's purpose, passions, and desires? Does the other meet you in the areas you want to be met? Is there mutuality and equality? Is there an active and conscious working toward this between you, or is it largely unconscious? The second part of your Sacred Relationship is knowing your partner's desires, what will fulfill him or her, and what lessons are in his or her life. Do you fit together?

Nothing lasts forever. This is why beloved God needs to be brought in to complete the trinity of your Sacred Relationship. She is eternal, and this is your journey, with a supporting cast of characters to help you realize this. If you can support another in this journey, and if he or she can support you, you have a wonderful base for your relating to fulfill its highest purpose and ultimate goal.

This third party of the Divine in your relating will only ever bring more love and more truth to you both, completing your humanity with an infinite love that you will rarely be able to sustain or live with your human partners alone. In this ever-deepening humility, we realize wholeness within. We no longer need our partner as a crutch, to fill a hole within us, and can be happy with him or her *and* without him or her. Yet we also know we do desire him or her, simply because we enjoy him or her, we enjoy our love, our meeting, our lovemaking, our sharing, our fun, and the spontaneous adventure of life taking us into the vast unknown.

In this trinity man and woman find their right places and roles with each other. Woman surrenders, man holds; woman receives, man guides; woman moves the Shakti, man is the pillar. And they swap at different times, to complete their own inner male and female.

In the old paradigm we wanted someone to live with, grow old with, to share the bills with, to have kids with, to make life here easier, to make the vastness of life more manageable: the other became a crutch of sorts. Look at your parents.

In the new paradigm, we do not need the other. We have our own money, our own emotional security formed from our own deep inner work, our own sovereignty, our own wholeness and aloneness we enjoy. We can live and die alone, and we choose to relate to others out of a truly informed freedom of choice and willingness to share—not out of desperation, loneliness, or sadness, but out of exuberance, fulfillment, and peace. This is the beginning of Sacred Relationship.

We live in our own personal web of life, a web in which all of our relationships inform each other. I found that being a father helped my own intimate relationship. I did not separate my different forms of relationship; I included them all. I would not settle for anything less, and this too benefited my partner. Sacred Relationship brings a total freedom of expression of all parts of you. Anything is allowed. Everything is permitted. All can be revealed for sharing, healing, and fun. The more honest you are, the more you release, the more whole you become.

You can be the child, the mother, the father, the wise grandfather, the raunchy woman, the primal man, the holy woman, and the holy man, and all parts are accepted and played out until there is no more to play with. You have embodied them all. Then you move into Sacred Relationship. Everything has to be seen and felt for this movement to occur. Do not leave even one single part of you out of this! Only you will lose out, not the other. Reveal all to have all. Give all to receive all.

One way we viscerally, palpably taste the goodness of this all-ness is through sacred union in lovemaking. When all of a woman's body, soul, and womb becomes one, throbbing, pulsating yoni, ripe and ready to be entered, juicy and surrendered, and all-attractive and magnetically alluring, a man cannot resist. This only happens when a man has embodied true forgiveness and all parts of him are united in honor, embodying the lingam pillar of light. When a man enters his partner from yoni through womb to heart, crown, and beyond into God, his partner becomes imbued, infused, permeated by Presence. She enters ecstasy and the void through her partner's pillar. This union is not just in the bedroom: it is felt much of the time. It is a union with your own soul *as well as* a union with the other, to lead you into the greatest union ever possible: union with beloved God.

This Trinity completes you as human, as Divine.

In this spirit, I wish you all the grace, all the humility, all the love, all the adventure, all the fun, all the sobering and stark moments that change your life, all the transformation that brings true meaning and new substance to you, and all the infinite love God wishes to give you, now and forever more.

NAMASTE!
PADMA AON PRAKASHA

INDEX